DIFFERENTIAL EQUATION ANALYSIS IN BIOMEDICAL SCIENCE AND ENGINEERING

DIFFERENTIAL EQUATION ANALYSIS IN BIOMEDICAL SCIENCE AND ENGINEERING

PARTIAL DIFFERENTIAL EQUATION APPLICATIONS WITH R

William E. Schiesser
Department of Chemical Engineering
Lehigh University
Bethlehem, PA

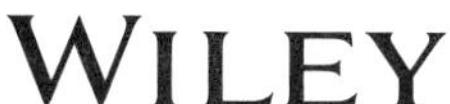

Cover Design: Wiley
Cover Illustration: Courtesy of the author

Published by John Wiley & Sons, Inc., Hoboken, New Jersey.
Published simultaneously in Canada.

Library of Congress Cataloging-in-Publication Data:

Schiesser, W. E.
Differential equation analysis in biomedical science and engineering : partial differential equation applications with R / William E. Schiesser, Department of Chemical Engineering, Lehigh University, Bethlehem, PA.
pages cm
Includes bibliographical references and index.
ISBN 978-1-118-70518-6 (cloth)
1. Biomedical engineering–Computer simulation. 2. Developmental biology–Simulation methods. 3. Chemotaxis–Data processing. 4. Differential equations. I. Title.
R857.M34.S345 2013
610.280285–dc23

2013020441

Printed in the United States of America.
10 9 8 7 6 5 4 3 2 1

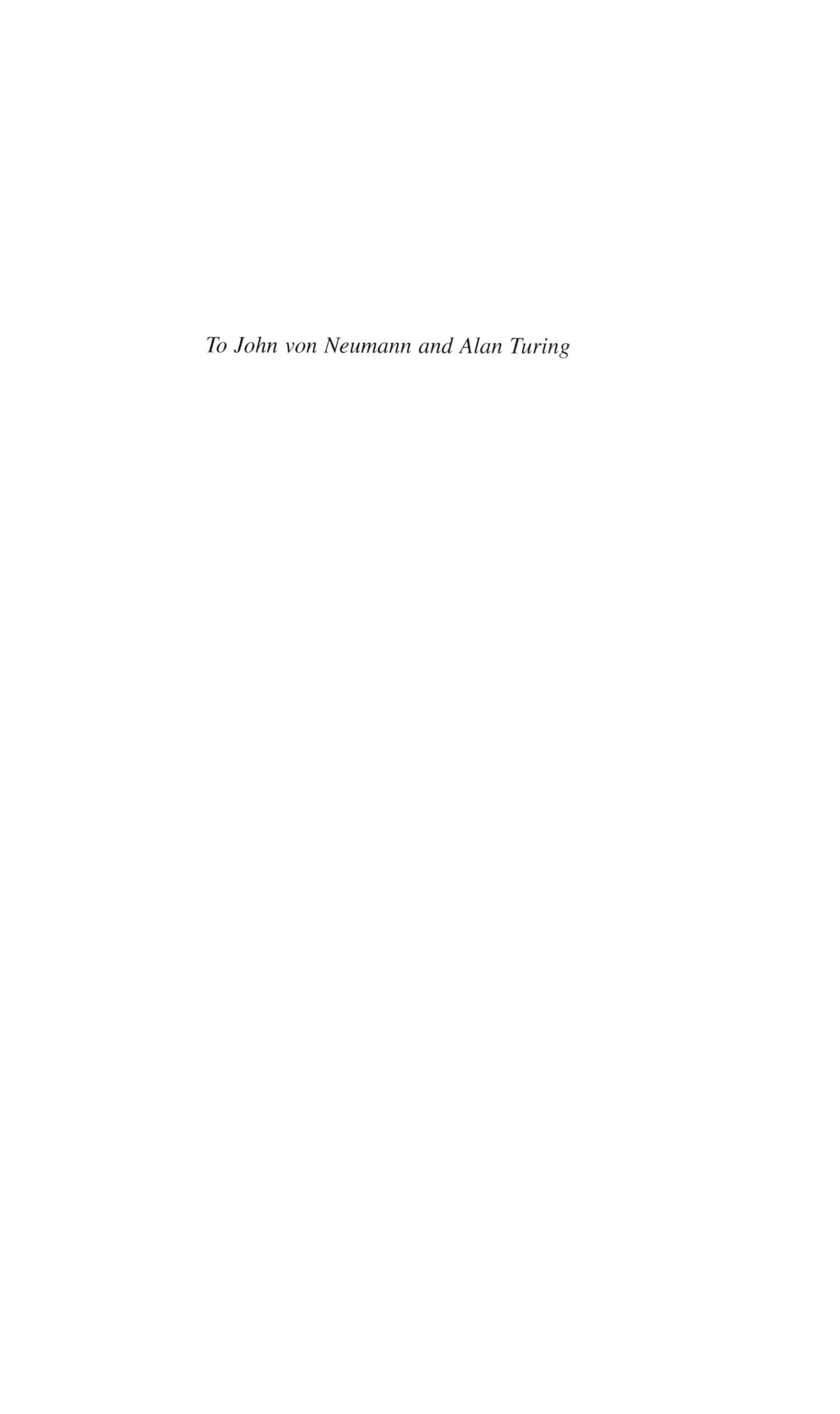

To John von Neumann and Alan Turing

CONTENTS

PREFACE

This book focuses on the rapidly expanding development and use of computer-based mathematical models in the life sciences, designated here as biomedical science and engineering (BMSE). The mathematical models are stated as systems of partial differential equations (PDEs) and generally come from papers in the current research literature that typically include the following steps:

1. The model is presented as a system of PDEs that explain associated chemistry, physics, biology, and physiology.
2. A numerical solution to the model equations is presented, particularly a discussion of the important features of the solution.

What is missing in this two-step approach are the details of how the solution was computed, particularly the details of the numerical algorithms. Also, because of the limited length of a research paper, the computer code used to produce the numerical solution is not provided. Thus, for the reader to reproduce (confirm) the solution and extend it is virtually impossible with reasonable effort.

The intent of this book is to fill in the steps for selected example applications that will give the reader the knowledge to reproduce and possibly extend the numerical solutions with reasonable effort. Specifically, the numerical algorithms are discussed in some detail, with additional background references, so that the reader will have some understanding of how the calculations were performed, and a set of transportable routines in R that the reader can study and execute to produce and extend the solutions is provided.[1]

Thus, the typical format of a chapter includes the following steps:

1. The model is presented as a system of PDEs that explain associated chemistry, physics, biology, and physiology. The requirements of a well-posed set of equations such as the number of dependent variables, the number of PDEs, algebraic equations used to calculate intermediate variables, and the initial and boundary conditions for the PDEs are included (which is often not the case in research papers so that all of the details of the model are not included or known to the reader).
2. The features of the model that determine the selection of numerical algorithms are discussed; for example, how spatial derivatives are approximated, whether the MOL ODEs are nonstiff or stiff, and therefore, whether an explicit or implicit integration algorithm has been used. The computational requirements of the particular selected algorithms are identified such as the solution of nonlinear equations, banded matrix processing, or sparse matrix processing.
3. The routines that are the programming of the PDEs and numerical algorithms are completely listed and then each section of code is explained, including referral to the mathematical model and the algorithms. Thus, all of the computational details for producing a numerical solution are in one place. Reference to another source for the software, possibly with little or no documentation, is thereby avoided.

[1]R is a quality open source scientific programming system that can be easily downloaded from the Internet (`http://www.R-project.org/`). In particular, R has (i) vector-matrix operations that facilitate the programming of linear algebra, (ii) a library of quality ODE integrators that can also be applied to PDE and ODE/PDE systems through the numerical method of lines (MOL), and (iii) graphical utilities for the presentation of the numerical solutions. All of these features and utilities are demonstrated through the applications in this book.

4. A numerical solution to the model equations is presented, particularly a discussion of the important features of the solution.
5. The accuracy of the computed solution is inferred using established methods such as h and p refinement. Alternative algorithms and computational details are considered, particularly to extend the model and the numerical solution.

In this way, a complete picture of the model and its computer implementation is provided without having to try to fill in the details of the numerical analysis, algorithms, and computer programming (often a time-consuming procedure that leads to an incomplete and unsatisfactory result). The presentation is not heavily mathematical, for example, no theorems and proofs, but rather the presentation is in terms of detailed examples of BMSE applications.

End of the chapter problems have not been provided. Rather, the instructor can readily construct problems and assignments that will be in accordance with the interests and objectives of the instructor. This can be done in several ways by developing variations and extensions of the applications discussed in the chapters. The following are a few examples.

1. Parameters in the model equations can be varied, and the effects on the computed solutions can be observed and explained. Exploratory questions can be posed such as whether the changes in the solutions are as expected. In addition, the terms in the right-hand sides (RHSs) of the PDEs (without the derivatives in the initial-value independent variable, usually time) can be computed and displayed numerically and graphically to explain in detail why the parameter changes had the observed effect. The computation and display of PDE RHS terms is illustrated in selected chapters to serve as a guide.
2. Additional terms can be added to the PDE RHSs to model physical, chemical, and biological effects that might be significant in determining the characteristics of the problem system. These additional terms can be computed and displayed along with the

original terms to observe which terms have a significant effect on the computed model solution.

3. One or more PDEs can be added to an existing model to include additional phenomena that are considered possibly relevant to the analysis and understanding of the problem system. Also, ODEs can be added, typically as boundary conditions.
4. An entirely new model can be proposed and programmed for comparison with an existing model. The existing routines might serve as a starting point, for example, as a template.

These suggested problem formats are in the order of increasing generality to encourage the reader to explore new directions, including the revision of an existing model and the creation of a new model. This process is facilitated through the availability of existing routines for a model that can first be executed and then modified. The trial-and-error development of a model can be explored, particularly if experimental data that can be used as the basis for model development are provided, starting from parameter estimation based on a comparison of experimentally measured data and computed solutions from an existing model, up to the development of a new model to interpret the data.

The focus of this book is primarily on models expressed as systems of PDEs that generally result from including spatial effects so that the dependent variables of the PDEs, for example, concentrations, are functions of space and time, which is a basic distinguishing characteristic of PDEs (ODEs have only one independent variable, typically time). The spatial derivatives require boundary conditions for a complete specification of the PDE model and several boundary condition types are discussed in the example applications.

In summary, my intention is to provide a set of basic computational procedures for ODE/PDE models that readers can use with modest effort without becoming deeply involved in the details of numerical methods for ODE/PDEs and computer programming. All of the R routines discussed in this PDE volume and the companion ODE volume *Differential Equation Analysis in Biomedical Science and Engineering: Ordinary Differential Equation Applications with R* are available from a software download site, booksupport.wiley.com, which requires the ISBN: 9781118705483 for the ODE volume or 9781118705186 for this volume. I welcome comments and will be pleased to respond to questions to the extent possible by e-mail (wes1@lehigh.edu).

William E. Schiesser

Bethlehem, PA
February 2014

CHAPTER 1

Introduction to Partial Differentiation Equation Analysis: Chemotaxis

1.1 Introduction

This chapter serves as an introduction to the analysis of biomedical science and engineering (BMSE) systems based on partial differential equations (PDEs) programmed in R. The general format of this chapter and the chapters that follow consists of the following steps:

- Presentation of a PDE model as a system of PDEs, possibly with the inclusion of some additional ordinary differential equations (ODEs).
- Review of algorithms for the numerical solution of the PDE model.
- Discussion of a set of R routines that implement the numerical algorithms as applied to the model.
- Review of the computed output.
- Conclusions concerning the model, computer implementation, output, and possible extensions of the analysis.

This format is introductory and application oriented with a minimum of mathematical formality. The intention is to help the reader

Differential Equation Analysis in Biomedical Science and Engineering: Partial Differential Equation Applications with R, First Edition. William E. Schiesser.

start with PDE analysis of BMSE systems without becoming deeply involved in the details of PDE numerical methods and their computer implementation (e.g., coding). Also, the presentation is self-contained so that the reader will not have to go to other sources such as a software download to find the routines that are discussed and used in a particular application. Our final objective then is for the detailed discussions of the various applications to facilitate a start in the PDE analysis of BMSE systems.

In this chapter, we consider the following topics.

- A brief introduction to PDEs.
- Application of PDE analysis to chemotaxis.
- Algorithms for the numerical solution of a simultaneous 2-PDE nonlinear chemotaxis model.
- Computer routines for implementation of the numerical algorithms.
- Traveling wave features of the 2-PDE chemotaxis model numerical solution.

1.2 Linear Diffusion Model

Inanimate systems have the general feature wherein chemical species move from regions of high concentration to regions of low concentration by mechanisms that are often modeled as diffusion, that is, according to Fick's first and second laws. In 1D, this diffusion is described (according to Fick's second law) as

$$\frac{\partial c}{\partial t} = \frac{\partial}{\partial x}\left[D\frac{\partial c}{\partial x}\right] \tag{1.1a}$$

where

c	volume concentration
x	spatial coordinate
t	time
D	diffusivity

In accordance with the usual convention for PDE notation, the dependent variable will subsequently be denoted as u rather than c. Thus, eq. (1.1a) will be

$$\frac{\partial u}{\partial t} = \frac{\partial}{\partial x}\left[D\frac{\partial u}{\partial x}\right] \tag{1.1a}$$

We can note the following features of eq. (1.1a).

- Eq. (1.1a) is a PDE because it has two independent variables, x and t. A differential equation with only one independent variable is termed an ordinary differential equation (ODE). Note also that ∂ is used to denote a partial derivative.
- The solution of eq. (1.1a) is the dependent variable u as a function of the independent variables x and t, that is, $u(x,t)$ in numerical form (rather than analytical form).
- Eq. (1.1a) is linear for constant D because the dependent variable u and its partial derivatives are to the first degree (not to be confused with order because eq. (1.1a) is first order in t because of the first-order derivative in t and second order in x because of the second-order derivative in x). Classifying eq. (1.1a) as linear presupposes that the diffusivity D is not a function of u. Eq. (1.1a) is nonlinear if $D = D(u)$ because of the product $D(u)\partial u/\partial x$.
- The diffusivity D is inside the first (left most) differentiation to handle the case when D is a function of x and/or u. If D is a constant, it can be moved outside the first differentiation.

Eq. (1.1a) models ordinary diffusion because of, for example, random motion of molecules. A distinguishing feature of this type of diffusion is net movement in the direction of decreasing concentration as reflected in Fick's first law

$$\mathbf{q}_x = -D\frac{\partial u}{\partial x} \tag{1.1b}$$

$\mathbf{q}_x$ is a component of the diffusion flux vector (with additional components $\mathbf{q}_y$ and $\mathbf{q}_z$ in Cartesian coordinates) and is therefore denoted with boldface. The minus sign signifies diffusion in the direction of decreasing concentration (as for $\partial u/\partial x < 0$, $\mathbf{q}_x > 0$).

Since eq. (1.1a) is first order in t and second order in x, it requires one initial condition (IC) and two boundary conditions (BCs). For example,

$$u(x,t=0) = f(x),\ 0 \le x \le x_L \tag{1.1c}$$

$$u(x=0,t) = g_1(t),\ u(x=x_L,t) = g_2(t),\ t > 0 \tag{1.1d,e}$$

where x_L is a constant (length) to be specified and f_1, g_1, g_2 are functions to be specified. Since BCs (1.1d,e) specify the dependent variable $u(x,t)$ at two particular (boundary) values of x, that is, $x = 0, x_L$, they are termed *Dirichlet BCs*. The derivatives in x can be specified as BCs, for example,

$$\frac{\partial u(x=0,t)}{\partial x} = g_3(t),\ \frac{\partial u(x=x_L,t)}{\partial x} = g_4(t) \tag{1.1f,g}$$

Eqs. (1.1f) and (1.1g) are termed *Neumann BCs*. Also, the dependent variable and its derivative can be specified at a boundary, for example,

$$-\frac{u(x=0,t)}{\partial x} + u(x=0,t) = g_5(t), \tag{1.1h}$$

$$\frac{u(x=x_L,t)}{\partial x} + u(x=x_L,t) = g_6(t) \tag{1.1i}$$

Eqs. (1.1h) and (1.1i) are termed third-type, Robin, or natural BCs. All of these various forms of BCs (eqs. (1.1d)–(1.1i)) are useful in applications.

Finally, note that t is defined over an open-ended interval or domain, $t > 0$, and is termed an initial value variable (typically time in an application). x is defined between two different (boundary) values in x, denoted here as $0, x_L$ or more generally x_0, x_L (typically physical boundaries in an application). However, the interval in x can be semi-infinite, for example, $-\infty < x \le 0$, $0 \le x \le \infty$ or fully infinite, $-\infty < x < \infty$.

1.3 Nonlinear Chemotaxis Model

Eqs. (1.1a) and (1.1b) can be extended to a nonlinear form of Fick's first and second laws. Also, we can consider more than one dependent variable, and we now consider two dependent variables $u_1(x,t)$ and $u_2(x,t)$ in place of just $u(x,t)$. The 2-PDE model for chemotaxis is ([2], p 68)

$$u_{1t} = -ku_2 \tag{1.2a}$$

$$u_{2t} = D\frac{\partial}{\partial x}\left[u_{2x} - 2\frac{u_2}{u_1}u_{1x}\right] \tag{1.2b}$$

Here, we have employed subscript notation for some of the partial derivatives. For example,

$$\frac{\partial u_1}{\partial t} \Rightarrow u_{1t}, \frac{\partial u_1}{\partial x} \Rightarrow u_{1x}, \frac{\partial u_2}{\partial t} \Rightarrow u_{2t}$$

Note that the PDE variables can have two subscripts. The first is a number denoting a particular dependent variable. The second is a letter denoting a partial derivative with respect to a particular independent variable. For example, u_{1t} denotes the first dependent variable u_1 differentiated with respect to t. Also, the second (letter) subscript can be repeated to denote a higher order derivative. For example, subscript notation can be used in eq. (1.2b),

$$\frac{\partial}{\partial x}[u_{2x}] = u_{2xx}$$

$$\frac{\partial}{\partial x}\left[-2\frac{u_2}{u_1}u_{1x}\right] = \left[-2\frac{u_2}{u_1}u_{1x}\right]_x$$

This compact subscript notation for partial derivatives can be useful in conveying a correspondence between the mathematics and the associated computer coding. This will be illustrated in the subsequent programming of eqs. (1.2).

The variables and parameters in eqs. (1.2) are

u_1	attractant concentration
u_2	bacteria concentration
x	spatial coordinate
t	time
k	rate constant
D	diffusivity

Eqs. (1.2) defines the volume concentration of a microorganism (such as bacteria), $u_2(x,t)$, when responding to an attractant (such as a nutrient or food supply), $u_1(x,t)$. Eq. (1.2a) reflects the rate of consumption of u_1, that is, u_{1t}, due to u_2; the rate constant is taken as $k > 0$ so that the minus is required for consumption ($u_{1t} \leq 0$ with $u_2 \geq 0$).

Eq. (1.2b) is an extension of eq. (1.1b) and implies a diffusion flux $\mathbf{q}$ in the x-direction.

$$\mathbf{q} = -D\left[u_{2x} - 2\frac{u_2}{u_1}u_{1x}\right] \tag{1.2c}$$

(the subscript x in $\mathbf{q}_x$ has been dropped). Eq. (1.2c) can be considered an extension of eq. (1.1b). It is nonlinear because of the term $(u_2/u_1)u_{1x}$. We can note the following details about eq. (1.2c).

- The first RHS term, $-Du_{2x}$, is just Fick's first law, eq. (1.1b). In other words, the flux of eq. (1.2c), $\mathbf{q}$, is composed partly of the usual flux in the direction of decreasing gradient ($Du_{2x} < 0$, which tends to make $\mathbf{q} > 0$ because of the minus sign in eq. (1.2c)).
- The second RHS term is opposite in sign to the first and, therefore, gives the opposite effect for the flux $\mathbf{q}$. Note that the gradient in this term is u_{1x}, not u_{2x}. Thus, this term causes the bacteria flux $\mathbf{q}$ to increase with increasing attractant concentration u_1. Also, the ratio u_2/u_1 is a factor in determining the flux $\mathbf{q}$. This ratio causes the rate of transfer (flux) of the bacteria, $\mathbf{q}$, to increase with increasing bacteria concentration, u_2, and also to increase with a decrease in the attractant concentration, u_1;

for the latter, the bacteria apparently move faster when facing decreasing availability of the attractant (e.g., nutrient or food). Clearly, this nonlinear RHS term is a significant departure from the diffusion term of Fick's first law, eq. (1.1b). This is a unique feature of chemotaxis by which the bacteria seek higher concentrations of the attractant; this seems plausible if, for example, the attractant is a nutrient such as food. This effect is clearly a feature of an animate (living) system, such as bacteria, rather than an inanimate system.

- As the second RHS term has a rather unconventional form, we would expect that it will introduce unusual features in the solution when compared with the usual diffusion modeled by Fick's first and second laws. These features will be considered when the routines for the solution of eqs. (1.2a) and (1.2b) are discussed subsequently.
- As the nonlinear diffusion term $-2D(u_2/u_1)u_{1x}$ requires $u_1(x,t)$, it is necessary to integrate eq. (1.2a) along with (1.2b); in other words, u_1 and u_{1x} come from eq. (1.2a). But the solution of eq. (1.2a) requires u_2 from eq. (1.2b) (in the RHS term of eq. (1.2a)). Thus, eqs. (1.2a) and (1.2b) must be integrated together to give $u_1(x,t)$ and $u_2(x,t)$ simultaneously. This requirement might be designated as a 2×2 system (two PDEs, eqs. (1.2a) and (1.2b), in two unknowns, u_1, u_2).

Eqs. (1.2a) and (1.2b) are first order in t and therefore each requires an IC

$$u_1(x,t=0) = f_1(x), \; u_2(x,t=0) = f_2(x) \tag{1.3a,b}$$

where f_1 and f_2 are functions to be specified.

Eq. (1.2b) is second order in x and, therefore, requires two BCs. As $u_1(x,t)$ is a function of x, and it appears in a second derivative term in eq. (1.2b), we will also assign it two BCs.

$$\frac{\partial u_1(x \to -\infty, t)}{\partial x} = \frac{\partial u_1(x \to \infty, t)}{\partial x} = 0 \tag{1.4a,b}$$

$$\frac{\partial u_2(x \to -\infty, t)}{\partial x} = \frac{\partial u_2(x \to \infty, t)}{\partial x} = 0 \tag{1.4c,d}$$

The analytical solution to eqs. (1.2)–(1.4) is ([2], p 68)

$$u_1(z) = [1 + e^{-cz/D}]^{-1} \tag{1.5a}$$

$$u_2(z) = \frac{c^2}{kD} e^{-cz/D}[1 + e^{-cz/D}]^{-2} \tag{1.5b}$$

where $z = x - ct$; c is a constant to be specified (a velocity). Note that $u_1(z)$ and $u_2(z)$ are a function of the single Lagrangian variable z. In other words, these solutions are invariant for a constant value of z, regardless of how x and t may vary. A solution with this property is termed a *traveling wave* [1]. We will discuss this property further when the numerical solution to eqs. (1.2) is discussed subsequently.

We will use eqs. (1.5) for ICs (1.3) with $t = 0, z = x$.

$$f_1(x) = u_1(x, t = 0) = [1 + e^{-cx/D}]^{-1} \tag{1.3c}$$

$$f_2(x) = u_2(x, t = 0) = \frac{c^2}{kD} e^{-cx/D}[1 + e^{-cx/D}]^{-2} \tag{1.3d}$$

Eqs. (1.2)–(1.4) constitute the 2-PDE model to be studied numerically. Also, the analytical solutions, eqs. (1.5), will be used to evaluate the numerical solution.

1.4 Method of Lines Solution of 2-PDE Chemotaxis Model

The method of lines (MOL) is a general procedure for the numerical integration of PDEs in which the derivatives in the boundary value (spatial) independent variables are approximated algebraically, in the present case, by finite differences (FDs). Then only one independent variable remains, in this case, the initial value t. As we have now only one independent variable, the original PDEs are replaced with an approximating set of ODEs. These ODEs can then be integrated (solved) numerically by any established initial value ODE integrator. In the discussion that follows, we will use the R ODE integrator `lsodes` [3]. This is the essence of the numerical MOL.

The R routines for PDEs (1.2), ICs (1.3), and BCs (1.4) follow. The numerical solution from these routines will then be compared with the analytical solution, eqs. (1.5). A main program for the numerical MOL solution is in Listing 1.1.

1.4.1 Main Program

The following main program is for eqs. (1.2), (1.3) and (1.4).

```
#
# Access ODE integrator
  library("deSolve");
#
# Access functions for analytical solutions
  setwd("c:/R/bme_pde/chap1");
  source("chemo_1.R");
  source("u1_anal.R");
  source("u2_anal.R");
  source("dss004.R");
#
# Level of output
#
#   ip = 1 - graphical (plotted) solutions
#            (u1(x,t), u2(x,t)) only
#
#   ip = 2 - numerical and graphical solutions
#
  ip=3;
#
# Grid (in x)
  nx=101;xl=-10;xu=15
  xg=seq(from=xl,to=xu,by=0.25);
#
# Parameters
  k=1;D=1;c=1;
  cat(sprintf("\n\n k = %5.2f   D = %5.2f   c = %5.2f\n",
     k,D,c));
#
# Independent variable for ODE integration
  nout=6;
  tout=seq(from=0,to=5,by=1);
#
# Initial condition (from analytical solutions,t=0)
  u0=rep(0,2*nx);
```

```
  for(i in 1:nx){
    u0[i]  =u1_anal(xg[i],tout[1],k,D,c);
    u0[i+n]=u2_anal(xg[i],tout[1],k,D,c);
  }
  ncall=0;
#
# ODE integration
  out=lsodes(y=u0,times=tout,func=chemo_1,parms=NULL)
  nrow(out)
  ncol(out)
#
# Arrays for plotting numerical, analytical solutions
  u1_plot=matrix(0,nrow=nx,ncol=nout);
  u2_plot=matrix(0,nrow=nx,ncol=nout);
 u1a_plot=matrix(0,nrow=nx,ncol=nout);
 u2a_plot=matrix(0,nrow=nx,ncol=nout);
  for(it in 1:nout){
    for(ix in 1:nx){
       u1_plot[ix,it]=out[it,ix+1];
       u2_plot[ix,it]=out[it,ix+1+nx];
      u1a_plot[ix,it]=u1_anal(xg[ix],tout[it],k,D,c);
      u2a_plot[ix,it]=u2_anal(xg[ix],tout[it],k,D,c);
    }
  }
#
# Display numerical solution
  if(ip==2){
    for(it in 1:nout){
      cat(sprintf("\n    t        x   u1(x,t)  u1_ex(x,t)
         u1_err(x,t)"));
      cat(sprintf("\n                      u2(x,t)  u2_ex(x,t)
         u2_err(x,t)\n"));
      for(ix in 1:nx){
        cat(sprintf("%5.1f%8.2f%10.5f%12.5f%13.6f\n",
           tout[it],xg[ix],
        u1_plot[ix,it],u1a_plot[ix,it],u1_plot[ix,it]-
           u1a_plot[ix,it]));
        cat(sprintf("             %10.5f%12.5f%13.6f\n",
        u2_plot[ix,it],u2a_plot[ix,it],u2_plot[ix,it]-
           u2a_plot[ix,it]));
      }
```

```
    }
  }
#
# Calls to ODE routine
  cat(sprintf("\n\n ncall = %5d\n\n",ncall));
#
# Plot u1 numerical, analytical
  par(mfrow=c(1,1));
  matplot(x=xg,y=u1_plot,type="l",xlab="x",
     ylab="u1(x,t), t=0,1,2,3,4,5", xlim=c(xl,xu),lty=1,
     main="u1(x,t); solid - num, points - anal;
        t=0,1,2,3,4,5;",lwd=2);
  matpoints(x=xg,y=u1a_plot,xlim=c(xl,xu),col="black",
     lwd=2)
#
# Plot u2 numerical, analytical
  par(mfrow=c(1,1));
  matplot(x=xg,y=u2_plot,type="l",xlab="x",
     ylab="u2(x,t), t=0,1,2,3,4,5", xlim=c(xl,xu),lty=1,
     main="u2(x,t), solid - num, points - anal;
        t=0,1,2,3,4,5;",lwd=2);
  matpoints(x=xg,y=u2a_plot,xlim=c(xl,xu),col="black",
     lwd=2)
```

Listing 1.1 Main program for the solution of eqs. (1.2).

We can note the following details about Listing 1.1.

- The library of ODE solvers, `deSolve` (with `lsodes` for the subsequent integration of the MOL ODEs), is accessed. Also, four files with the routines to calculate the numerical and analytical solutions of eqs. (1.2) are accessed. Note the use of the forward slash / in `setwd` (set working directory).

```
#
# Access ODE integrator
  library("deSolve");
#
# Access functions for analytical solutions
  setwd("c:/R/bme_pde/chap1");
```

```
  source("chemo_1.R");
  source("u1_anal.R");
  source("u2_anal.R");
  source("dss004.R");
```

- Two cases are programmed: `ip=1` for graphical output only and `ip=2` for graphical and numerical outputs.

```
#
# Level of output
#
#   ip = 1 - graphical (plotted) solutions
#            (u1(x,t), u2(x,t)) only
#
#   ip = 2 - numerical and graphical solutions
#
  ip=2;
```

- A grid in x is defined over the interval $-10 \leq x \leq 15$ with `nx=101` points. This x domain was selected to be essentially infinite as required by BCs (1.4). This characteristic will be explained later. `101` points were determined to be adequate to achieve acceptable accuracy (spatial resolution), and this accuracy is confirmed by comparing the numerical solution to the analytical solution of eqs. (1.5).

```
#
# Grid (in x)
  nx=101;xl=-10;xu=15
  xg=seq(from=xl,to=xu,by=0.25);
```

- The model parameters (constants) are defined numerically and displayed. These parameters appear in eqs. (1.2) and (1.5).

```
#
# Parameters
  k=1;D=1;c=1;
  cat(sprintf("\n\n k = %5.2f   D = %5.2f   c =
     %5.2f\n",k,D,c));
```

- Six output values of t are placed in vector `tout`, that is, `tout=0,1,2,3,4,5`.

```
#
# Independent variable for ODE integration
  nout=6;
  tout=seq(from=0,to=5,by=1);
```

A total of six outputs (counting the IC) provides parametric plots in t (for $t = 0, 1, \ldots, 5$) as explained subsequently.

- The ICs of eqs. (1.3) are computed from the analytical solutions of eqs. (1.5) with t = `tout[1]` = 0 (in routines `u1_anal,u2_anal`) and placed in a single vector `u0` for subsequent use as an input to the ODE integrator `lsodes` to start the numerical solution.

```
#
# Initial condition (from analytical solutions,t=0)
  u0=rep(0,2*nx);
  for(i in 1:nx){
    u0[i]   =u1_anal(xg[i],tout[1],k,D,c);
    u0[i+nx]=u2_anal(xg[i],tout[1],k,D,c);
  }
  ncall=0;
```

Note that there are `2*nx = 2*101` = 202 ICs and MOL ODEs that approximate the PDEs, eqs. (1.2). The length of `u0` informs the ODE integrator, `lsodes`, of the number of ODEs to be integrated (`202`). The counter for the calls to the ODE routine (discussed subsequently) is also initialized.

- The integration of the 202 ODEs is accomplished by a call to `lsodes`.

```
#
# ODE integration
  out=lsodes(y=u0,times=tout,func=chemo_1,parms=NULL)
  nrow(out)
  ncol(out)
```

We can note the following details about the call to `lsodes`.

- The IC vector `u0` is used to start the ODE integration (the parameter `y` is a reserved name for `lsodes`).

- The output values of t are in vector tout defined previously. These values of t are also returned through the 2D solution array out (times is a reserved name for lsodes).
- The ODE routine chemo_1 discussed subsequently is used for the calculation of the 202 ODE derivatives (func is a reserved name for lsodes).
- The parameter parms is unused. It could pass the parameters k,D,c to chemo_1 but these parameters are already global (a feature of R) and therefore are available in chemo_1 (parms is a reserved name for lsodes).
- The ODE solution is returned in a 2D array out. In other words, all $n = 202$ ODE solutions are returned in out at each of the nout=6 values of t. However, the dimensions of out are out(6,203) with an additional value in the second dimension (203 rather than 202) for t. This dimensioning of out is confirmed by the R utilities nrow,ncol; note that if a concluding ; is not used in calling nrow,ncol, the numerical values of the number of rows and columns (6,203) are displayed.

- The ODE solution returned in out is placed in two 2D arrays, u1_plot,u2_plot.

```
#
# Arrays for plotting numerical, analytical solutions
  u1_plot=matrix(0,nrow=nx,ncol=nout);
  u2_plot=matrix(0,nrow=nx,ncol=nout);
 u1a_plot=matrix(0,nrow=nx,ncol=nout);
 u2a_plot=matrix(0,nrow=nx,ncol=nout);
  for(it in 1:nout){
    for(ix in 1:nx){
       u1_plot[ix,it]=out[it,ix+1];
       u2_plot[ix,it]=out[it,ix+1+nx];
      u1a_plot[ix,it]=u1_anal(xg[ix],tout[it],k,D,c);
      u2a_plot[ix,it]=u2_anal(xg[ix],tout[it],k,D,c);
    }
  }
```

Also, the analytical solutions of eqs. (1.5) are placed in two 2D arrays, u1a_plot and u2a_plot so that the numerical and analytical solutions can be compared. The routines for the analytical solutions, u1_anal and u2_anal, are discussed subsequently. Note the offset of 1 in the second subscript of out, for example, ix+1. This offset is required because the first value of this subscript is used for the values of t, that is, out[it,1] has the values $t = 0, 1, 2, 3, 5$ corresponding to it=1,2,...,6 (this is a property of the numerical solution in out from lsodes).

- For ip=2, the numerical solution is displayed in a tabulated format (Table 1.1).

```
#
# Display numerical solution
  if(ip==2){
    for(it in 1:nout){
      cat(sprintf("\n     t        x    u1(x,t)   u1_ex
         (x,t)    u1_err(x,t)"));
      cat(sprintf("\n                       u2(x,t)   u2_ex
         (x,t)    u2_err(x,t)\n"));
      for(ix in 1:nx){
        cat(sprintf("%5.1f%8.2f%10.5f%12.5f%13.6f\n",
           tout[it],xg[ix],
        u1_plot[ix,it],u1a_plot[ix,it],u1_plot[ix,it]
           -u1a_plot[ix,it]));
        cat(sprintf("             %10.5f%12.5f%
           13.6f\n",
        u2_plot[ix,it],u2a_plot[ix,it],u2_plot[ix,it]
           -u2a_plot[ix,it]));
      }
    }
  }
```

- The number of calls to chemo_1 is displayed at the end of the solution.

```
#
# Calls to ODE routine
  cat(sprintf("\n\n ncall = %5d\n\n",ncall));
```

- $u_1(x,t)$ and $u_2(x,t)$ are plotted against x with t as a parameter in Figs. 1.1 and 1.2.

```
#
# Plot u1 numerical, analytical
  par(mfrow=c(1,1));
  matplot(x=xg,y=u1_plot,type="l",xlab="x",
    ylab="u1(x,t), t=0,1,...,5",xlim=c(xl,xu),lty=1,
    main="u1(x,t); t=0,1,...,5; lines - num, points -
       anal",lwd=2);
  matpoints(x=xg,y=u1a_plot,xlim=c(xl,xu),col="black",
      lwd=2)
#
# Plot u2 numerical, analytical
  par(mfrow=c(1,1));
  matplot(x=xg,y=u2_plot,type="l",xlab="x",
    ylab="u2(x,t), t=0,1,...,5",xlim=c(xl,xu),lty=1,
    main="u2(x,t), t=0,1,...,5; lines - num, points -
       anal",lwd=2);
  matpoints(x=xg,y=u2a_plot,xlim=c(xl,xu),col="black",
      lwd=2)
```

`par(mfrow=c(1,1))` specifies a 1×1 array of plots, that is, a single plot. The R utility `matplot` plots the 2D array with the numerical solutions, `u1_plot,u2_plot`, and the utility `matpoints` superimposes the analytical solutions in `u1a_plot` and `u2a_plot` as points. These details plus the others specified with the various arguments (e.g., axis labels, x axis limits, main heading) are clear when considering Figs. 1.1 and 1.2.

We now consider the routines called by the main program of Listing 1.1, starting with `chemo_1`. The numerical and graphical output from Listing 1.1 is then considered.

1.4.2 ODE Routine

The ODE routine for the MOL solution of eqs. (1.2) follows.

```
  chemo_1=function(t,u,parms){
#
# Function chemo_1 computes the t derivative vectors of
   u1(x,t), u2(x,t)
#
# One vector to two vectors
```

```
  u1=rep(0,nx);u2=rep(0,nx);
  for(i in 1:nx){
    u1[i]=u[i];
    u2[i]=u[i+nx];
  }
#
# u1x, u2x
  u1x=rep(0,nx);u2x=rep(0,nx);
  u1x=dss004(xl,xu,nx,u1);
  u2x=dss004(xl,xu,nx,u2);
#
# BCs
  u1x[1]=0; u1x[nx]=0;
  u2x[1]=0; u2x[nx]=0;
#
# Nonlinear term
  u1u2x=rep(0,nx);
  for(i in 1:nx){
    u1u2x[i]=2*u2[i]/u1[i]*u1x[i];
  }
#
# u1u2xx, u2xx
  u2xx=rep(0,nx);u1u2xx=rep(0,nx);
  u2xx  =dss004(xl,xu,nx,  u2x);
  u1u2xx=dss004(xl,xu,nx,u1u2x);
#
# PDEs
  u1t=rep(0,nx);u2t=rep(0,nx);
  for(i in 1:nx){
    u1t[i]=-k*u2[i];
    u2t[i]=D*(u2xx[i]-u1u2xx[i]);
  }
#
# Two vectors to one vector
  ut=rep(0,2*nx);
  for(i in 1:nx){
    ut[i]   =u1t[i];
    ut[i+nx]=u2t[i];
  }
#
# Increment calls to chemo_1
```

```
  ncall <<- ncall+1;
#
# Return derivative vector
  return(list(c(ut)));
  }
```

Listing 1.2 ODE routine `chemo_1` called by the main program of Listing 1.1.

We can note the following details about Listing 1.2.

- The function is defined.

```
  chemo_1=function(t,u,parms){
#
# Function chemo_1 computes the t derivative vectors
   of u1(x,t), u2(x,t)
```

  The three input arguments are required by `lsodes`, which calls `chemo_1` (even though `parms` is not used). `u` is the input vector of the 202 dependent variables of ODE. `t` is the current value of the independent variable t.

- The single solution vector `u` is placed in two vectors `u1` and `u2` to facilitate the programming in terms of the dependent variables of eqs. (1.2).

```
#
# One vector to two vectors
  u1=rep(0,nx);u2=rep(0,nx);
  for(i in 1:nx){
    u1[i]=u[i];
    u2[i]=u[i+nx];
  }
```

- The first derivatives of `u1,u2` with respect to `x` are computed by calls to the library differentiator `dss004`.

```
#
# u1x, u2x
  u1x=rep(0,nx);u2x=rep(0,nx);
```

```
u1x=dss004(xl,xu,nx,u1);
u2x=dss004(xl,xu,nx,u2);
```

The boundary values of x, `xl=-10,xu=15`, are set in Listing 1.1 and are effectively for the interval $-\infty \leq x \leq \infty$.

- BCs (1.4) are programmed at `xl=-10,xu=15`. Note that this interval is not symmetric with respect to $x = 0$ because of the movement of the traveling wave solutions of eqs. (1.5) in the positive x-direction so that more distance is required for $x > 0$ than for $x < 0$. This feature of the interval in x will be clear when the numerical solution is examined graphically (plotted).

```
#
# BCs
  u1x[1]=0; u1x[nx]=0;
  u2x[1]=0; u2x[nx]=0;
```

The first derivatives of $u1$ and $u2$ are set to zero at the boundaries according to BCs (1.4).

- The nonlinear term in eqs. (1.2b) and (1.2c), $2(u_2/u_1)u_{1x}$, is computed and placed in array `u1u2x`

```
#
# Nonlinear term
  u1u2x=rep(0,nx);
  for(i in 1:nx){
    u1u2x[i]=2*u2[i]/u1[i]*u1x[i];
  }
```

- The second derivatives in eq. (1.2b) are computed by `dss004`. The calculation of the second derivative as the derivative of the first derivative is termed *stagewise differentiation*. This procedure is put to good use to calculate the derivative of the nonlinear term $2(u_2/u_1)u_{1x}$. This demonstrates a major advantage of the numerical solution of PDEs, that is, nonlinear terms of virtually any form can be accommodated.

```
#
# u1u2xx, u2xx
  u2xx=rep(0,nx);u1u2xx=rep(0,nx);
  u2xx  =dss004(xl,xu,nx,  u2x);
  u1u2xx=dss004(xl,xu,nx,u1u2x);
```

- Eqs. (1.2) are programmed

```
#
# PDEs
  u1t=rep(0,nx);u2t=rep(0,nx);
  for(i in 1:nx){
    u1t[i]=-k*u2[i];
    u2t[i]=D*(u2xx[i]-u1u2xx[i]);
  }
```

Note the resemblance of this programming to the PDEs (eqs. (1.2a) and (1.2b)), which is an important advantage of the MOL approach to the numerical solution of PDEs. If the term `-u1u2xx[i]` is not included, the resulting PDE `u2t[i]=D*(u2xx[i])` is just Fick's second law, eq. (1.1a) (with constant `D`).

- The two derivative vectors `u1t` and `u2t` are placed in a single derivative vector `ut` to be returned from `chemo_1`.

```
#
# Two vectors to one vector
  ut=rep(0,2*nx);
  for(i in 1:nx){
    ut[i]   =u1t[i];
    ut[i+nx]=u2t[i];
  }
```

- The counter for the calls to `chemo_1` is incremented (and returned to the main program with `<<-`).

```
#
# Increment calls to chemo_1
  ncall <<- ncall+1;
```

- The derivative vector `ut` is returned to `lsodes` as a list (a requirement of `lsodes`).

```
#
# Return derivative vector
  return(list(c(ut)));
  }
```

The final `}` concludes `chemo_1`.

In summary, chemo_1 receives the independent variable t and the dependent variable vector u (of length 2(101) = 202) as RHS (input) arguments and returns a derivative vector ut. Note that u and ut must be of the same length and the derivative of a particular dependent variable u[i] must be in position ut[i] in vector ut.

The straightforward coding in chemo_1 demonstrates the versatility of the MOL solution of eqs. (1.2), a 2×2 system of simultaneous nonlinear PDEs. Extensions to more complex PDE systems follows directly from the ideas expressed in chemo_1.

To complete the discussion of the R routines, we consider u1_anal and u2_anal for the analytical solutions of eqs. (1.5) (u1_anal and u2_anal are called in the main program of Listing 1.1 for numerical definition of the ICs of eqs. (1.3) and plotting of the analytical solutions (1.5)).

```
  u1_anal=function(x,t,k,D,c){
#
# Function u1_anal computes the analytical solution for
#    u1(x,t)
#
  z=x-c*t;
  u1a=1/(1+exp(-c*z/D));
#
# Return solution
  return(c(u1a));
  }
```

Listing 1.3a Routine u1_anal for the analytical solution of eq. (1.5a).

The programming of eq. (1.5a) in u1_anal is straightforward. We can note two details.

- The use of the Lagrangian variable z=x-c*t so that the solution is invariant for a particular value of z even though x and t vary. This produces a traveling wave solution as demonstrated in the graphical output described next.
- The value of the solution, u1a, is returned to the calling program—in this case, the main program of Listing 1.1—as a numerical vector (with one element, i.e., as a scalar). This

contrasts with chemo_1 in Listing 1.2 for which the derivative vector is returned as a list (as required by lsodes).

Function u2_anal is similar to u1_anal and follows directly from eq. (1.5b).

```
  u2_anal=function(x,t,k,D,c){
#
# Function u2_anal computes the analytical solution for
#    u2(x,t)
#
  z=x-c*t;
  u2a=(c^2/(k*D))*exp(-c*z/D)/(1+exp(-c*z/D))^2;
#
# Return solution
  return(c(u2a));
  }
```

Listing 1.3b Routine u2_anal for the analytical solution of eq. (1.5b).

This completes the programming of eqs. (1.2) with the associated ICs of eqs. (1.3) and the BCs of eqs. (1.4). We now consider the output from the routines in Listings 1.1–1.3.

1.5 Model Output

Execution of the main program in Listing 1.1 with ip=2 gives the abbreviated numerical output.

We can note the following details of the numerical output in Table 1.1.

- The model parameters are displayed.

```
k =   1.00    D =   1.00    c =   1.00
```

- The dimensions of the output array from lsodes are out[6, 203] as explained previously.

```
> nrow(out)
[1] 6
```

TABLE 1.1 Selected numerical output from the routines of Listings 1.1–1.3.

```
k =  1.00   D =  1.00   c =  1.00

> nrow(out)
[1] 6
> ncol(out)
[1] 203

  Output for t=0,1,2,3,4 removed

   t       x   u1(x,t)  u1_ex(x,t)  u1_err(x,t)
               u2(x,t)  u2_ex(x,t)  u2_err(x,t)
 5.0  -10.00   0.00000     0.00000     0.000001
               0.00000     0.00000     0.000003
 5.0   -9.75   0.00000     0.00000     0.000001
               0.00000     0.00000     0.000003
 5.0   -9.50   0.00000     0.00000     0.000001
               0.00000     0.00000     0.000003
 5.0   -9.25   0.00000     0.00000     0.000001
               0.00000     0.00000     0.000003
 5.0   -9.00   0.00000     0.00000     0.000001
               0.00000     0.00000     0.000003
                 .           .
                 .           .
                 .           .
     Output for x = -8.75 to 3.75 removed
                 .           .
                 .           .
                 .           .
 5.0    4.00   0.26894     0.26894    -0.000003
               0.19657     0.19661    -0.000044
 5.0    4.25   0.32081     0.32082    -0.000007
               0.21787     0.21789    -0.000029
 5.0    4.50   0.37754     0.37754    -0.000006
               0.23500     0.23500    -0.000009
 5.0    4.75   0.43782     0.43782     0.000001
               0.24614     0.24613     0.000009
```

(continued)

TABLE 1.1 *(Continued)*

```
5.0     5.00   0.50001      0.50000       0.000010
               0.25002      0.25000       0.000018
5.0     5.25   0.56220      0.56218       0.000019
               0.24615      0.24613       0.000013
5.0     5.50   0.62248      0.62246       0.000024
               0.23500      0.23500       0.000000
5.0     5.75   0.67920      0.67918       0.000024
               0.21788      0.21789      -0.000015
5.0     6.00   0.73108      0.73106       0.000019
               0.19659      0.19661      -0.000025
                  .            .
                  .            .
                  .            .
      Output for x = 6.25 to 13.75 removed
                  .            .
                  .            .
                  .            .
5.0    14.00   0.99986      0.99988      -0.000016
               0.00014      0.00012       0.000017
5.0    14.25   0.99988      0.99990      -0.000021
               0.00012      0.00010       0.000021
5.0    14.50   0.99990      0.99993      -0.000027
               0.00010      0.00007       0.000027
5.0    14.75   0.99991      0.99994      -0.000035
               0.00009      0.00006       0.000035
5.0    15.00   0.99991      0.99995      -0.000044
               0.00009      0.00005       0.000045

ncall =    295
```

```
> ncol(out)
[1] 203
```

In particular, the second dimension of `out` is `203` rather than `2*101` $= 202$ in order to include the value of t.

- The output for $t = 0, 1, 2, 3, 4$ is deleted to conserve space. Abbreviated output for $t = 5$ is displayed. In particular, the output for $x = 4$ to $x = 6$ demonstrates the following properties of the numerical and analytical solutions.

- For $x = 5, t = 5$, with $c = 1$, the Lagrangian variable is $z = x - ct = 5 - (1)(5) = 0$. For this value of z, the numerical and analytical solutions for `u1(x,t)` and `u2(x,t)` have the following values.

```
5.0     5.00    0.50001       0.50000       0.000010
                0.25002       0.25000       0.000018
```

  The numerical solution for `u1(x=5,t=5)` $= 0.50001$, whereas the analytical solution for `u1(x=5,t=5)` $= 0.50000$. Similarly, the numerical solution for `u2(x=5,t=5)` $= 0.25002$, whereas the analytical solution for `u2(x=5,t=5)` $= 0.25000$. This agreement between the numerical and analytical solutions is particularly noteworthy because at `x=5,t=5`, `u1(x,t)` and `u2(x,t)` are changing most rapidly (i.e., $z = 0$). In particular, `u2(x,t)` goes through a maximum with rapid change as indicated in Fig. 1.2.
- The computational effort to produce the numerical solution is modest.

```
ncall =  295
```

The plotted output from Listing 1.1 follows as Figs. 1.1 and 1.2. We can note the following details about Figs. 1.1 and 1.2.

- The agreement between the numerical (solid line) and the analytical solution of eq. (1.5a) (numbers) is quite satisfactory (as confirmed by Table 1.1). Thus, the grid with `nx=101` points appears to give acceptable spatial resolution in x. Of course, the number of grid points could be changed and the effect on the numerical solution of Table 1.1 could then be observed, a form of h refinement (because h is often used to denote the grid spacing in the numerical analysis literature). An alternative for evaluating the solution would be to compare the solution from `dss004` in `chemo_1` (based on five-point fourth-order FDs) with, for example, the solution from `dss006` (based on seven-point sixth-order FDs). This is a form of p refinement because p is

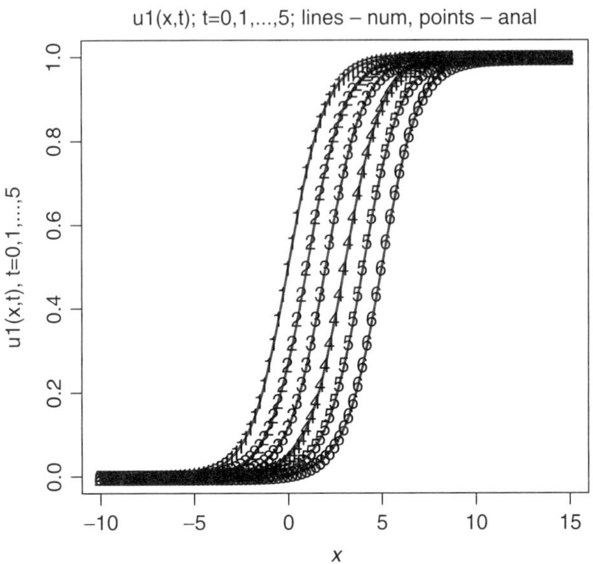

Figure 1.1 $u_1(x,t)$ versus x with t as a parameter.

often used to denote the order of an approximation; in the case of dss004 and dss006, $p = 4, 6$, respectively.

- The boundary values $x = -10, 15$ appear to be effectively at $-\infty, \infty$ in the sense that the solution does not change near these boundaries (note the zero derivative conditions of BCs (1.4)).
- The traveling wave characteristic of eqs. (1.2) and (1.5) is clear. That is, the solution moves left to right with a velocity $c = 1$ (in $z = x - ct$); the curves are for the six values $t = 0, 1, \ldots, 5$. The previous use of *characteristic* is more mathematical than might be appreciated. The Lagrangian variable $z = x - ct$ is generally termed a characteristic of the solution, and for a constant value of z, the solution is invariant; for example, the RHSs of eqs. (1.5) are invariant for a given value of z even though x and t may change.

In conclusion, the MOL solutions from the R routines in Listings 1.1–1.3 are in good agreement with the analytical solutions of

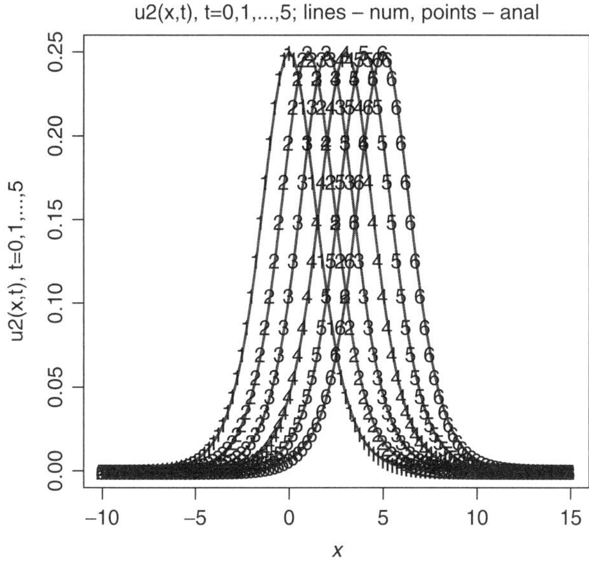

Figure 1.2 $u_2(x,t)$ versus x with t as a parameter.

eqs. (1.5). We now consider some additional programming to elucidate the origin of the solution properties in Table 1.1 and Figs. 1.1 and 1.2.

1.6 Computation of PDE Terms

One approach to understanding the solutions in Figs. 1.1 and 1.2 would be to derive an analytical solution such as eqs. (1.5) and then study these solutions mathematically. While this approach was possible in the case of eqs. (1.2)–(1.4), generally, the PDE problems that are studied numerically are so complex (e.g., too many nonlinear PDEs) as to preclude an analytical approach. We, therefore, consider a numerical approach to PDE analysis that can generally be used without an analytical solution but, rather, requires only the numerical solution.

Specifically, we consider PDEs such as eqs. (1.2) that have LHS terms that are functions of the derivatives in the initial value variable t and RHS terms that are functions of the derivatives in the spatial (boundary value) variable x (there could be more than one spatial variable). Then, a detailed examination of the RHS terms gives an indication of the mathematical details that define the variation of the dependent variables of PDE (the PDE solutions) with x. Also, a summation of the RHS terms according to the PDE gives an indication of the details of the LHS that define the variation of the numerical solutions with t. The only requirement to do this analysis in x and t is the availability of the numerical solution.

We now consider how this approach can be applied to eqs. (1.2)–(1.4) as an example of the detailed analysis of PDE numerical solutions. The programming for this analysis is the following code that is added to the end of Listing 1.1; nothing else changes in Listing 1.1 except the addition of a third value of the output index `ip`, that is, `ip=3`, to initiate the execution of the following code.

```
#
# Plotting of PDE RHS terms
  if(ip==3){
#
# 1D arrays of various PDE RHS terms (denoted 1d)
  u1_1d   =rep(0,nx); u2_1d =rep(0,nx);u1u2_1d=rep(0,nx);
  u1x_1d  =rep(0,nx);u2x_1d =rep(0,nx);
  u1u2x_1d=rep(0,nx);u2xx_1d=rep(0,nx);
#
# 2D arrays for plotting (denoted 2d)
  u1x_2d  =matrix(0,nrow=nx,ncol=nout);
  u2x_2d  =matrix(0,nrow=nx,ncol=nout);
  u1u2_2d =matrix(0,nrow=nx,ncol=nout);
  u2xx_2d =matrix(0,nrow=nx,ncol=nout);
  u1u2x_2d=matrix(0,nrow=nx,ncol=nout);
  u1t_2d  =matrix(0,nrow=nx,ncol=nout);
  u2t_2d  =matrix(0,nrow=nx,ncol=nout);
  u1x_2d_anal=matrix(0,nrow=nx,ncol=nout);
  u2x_2d_anal=matrix(0,nrow=nx,ncol=nout);
  u1t_2d_anal=matrix(0,nrow=nx,ncol=nout);
  u2t_2d_anal=matrix(0,nrow=nx,ncol=nout);
#
# PDE RHS terms
  for(it in 1:nout){
    for(ix in 1:nx){
      u1_1d[ix]=u1_plot[ix,it];
```

```
      u2_1d[ix]=u2_plot[ix,it];
    }
    u1x_1d=dss004(xl,xu,nx,u1_1d);
    u2x_1d=dss004(xl,xu,nx,u2_1d);
    u1x_1d[1]=0;u1x_1d[nx]=0;
    u2x_1d[1]=0;u2x_1d[nx]=0;
    for(ix in 1:nx){
      u1u2_1d[ix]=u2_1d[ix]/u1_1d[ix]*u1x_1d[ix];
    }
    u1u2x_1d=dss004(xl,xu,nx,u1u2_1d);
     u2xx_1d=dss004(xl,xu,nx, u2x_1d);
#
#   2D arrays for plotting
    for(ix in 1:n){
#
#     Derivatives of solutions in x
      u1x_2d[ix,it]=u1x_1d[ix];
      u2x_2d[ix,it]=u2x_1d[ix];
      u1u2_2d[ix,it]=u1u2_1d[ix];
      u2xx_2d[ix,it]=u2xx_1d[ix];
      u1u2x_2d[ix,it]=u1u2x_1d[ix];
#
#     Derivatives of solutions in t
      u1t_2d[ix,it]=-k*u2_1d[ix];
      u2t_2d[ix,it]=D*(u2xx_1d[ix]-2*u1u2x_1d[ix]);
#
#     Analytical derivatives of solutions in t
      expz=exp(-c*(xg[ix]-c*tout[it])/D);
      u1x_2d_anal[ix,it] =(1/c)*(1/(1+expz)^2)*expz*
         (c^2/D);
      u2x_2d_anal[ix,it]=-(1/c)* (c^4/(k*D^2))*expz*
         (1-expz)/(1+expz)^3;
      u1t_2d_anal[ix,it]=-c*u1x_2d_anal[ix,it];
      u2t_2d_anal[ix,it]=-c*u2x_2d_anal[ix,it];
    }
#
# Next t
  }
#
# Plot Du2_{xx}
  par(mfrow=c(1,1));
```

```
  matplot(x=xg,y=D*u2xx_2d,type="l",xlab="x",
     ylab="Du2_{xx},t=0,1,2,3,4,5",xlim=c(xl,xu),
        lty=1,main="Du2_{xx};t=0,1,2,3,4,5;",lwd=2);
#
# Plot -2D((u2/u1)u1_x)_x
  par(mfrow=c(1,1));
  matplot(x=xg,y=-2*D*u1u2x_2d,type="l",xlab="x",ylab=
     "-2D((u2/u1)u1_x)_x,t=0,1,2,3,4,5",xlim=c(xl,xu),
        lty=1,main="-2D((u2/u1)u1_x)_x,;t=0,1,2,3,4,5;",
           lwd=2);
#
# Plot u1 derivative in x numerical, analytical
  par(mfrow=c(1,1));
  matplot(x=xg,y=u1x_2d,type="l",xlab="x",ylab="u1(x,t)_x,
     t=0,1,2,3,4,5",xlim=c(xl,xu),lty=1,main="u1(x,t)_x;
        solid - num, points - anal;t=0,1,2,3,4,5;",
           lwd=2);
  matpoints(x=xg,y=u1x_2d_anal,xlim=c(xl,xu),col="black",
     lwd=2)
#
# Plot u2 derivative in x numerical, analytical
  par(mfrow=c(1,1));
  matplot(x=xg,y=u2x_2d,type="l",xlab="x",ylab="u2(x,t)_t,
     t=0,1,2,3,4,5",xlim=c(xl,xu),lty=1,main="u2(x,t)_x,
        solid - num, points - anal;t=0,1,2,3,4,5;",
           lwd=2);
  matpoints(x=xg,y=u2x_2d_anal,xlim=c(xl,xu),col="black",
     lwd=2)
#
# Plot u1 derivative in t numerical, analytical
  par(mfrow=c(1,1));
  matplot(x=xg,y=u1t_2d,type="l",xlab="x",ylab="u1(x,t)_t,
     t=0,1,2,3,4,5",xlim=c(xl,xu),lty=1,main="u1(x,t)_t;
        solid - num, points - anal;t=0,1,2,3,4,5;",
           lwd=2);
  matpoints(x=xg,y=u1t_2d_anal,xlim=c(xl,xu),col="black",
     lwd=2)
#
# Plot u2 derivative in t numerical, analytical
```

```
  par(mfrow=c(1,1));
  matplot(x=xg,y=u2t_2d,type="l",xlab="x",ylab="u2(x,t)_t,
     t=0,1,2,3,4,5",xlim=c(xl,xu),lty=1,main="u2(x,t)_t,
        solid - num, points - anal;t=0,1,2,3,4,5;",
           lwd=2);
  matpoints(x=xg,y=u2t_2d_anal,xlim=c(xl,xu),col="black",
     lwd=2)
#
# End ip = 3
  }
```

Listing 1.4 Additional programming to study the individual terms of eqs. (1.2).

We can note the following details of Listing 1.4.

- The execution of the code for `ip=3` is initiated with an `if`. Then, seven 1D arrays (vectors) are defined via the `rep` utility (these arrays are identified with `1d` in the names). The length of each vector equals the number of points in x, that is, `nx`, which is the length of vector `xg` in Listing 1.1.

```
#
# Plotting of PDE RHS terms
  if(ip==3){
#
# 1D arrays of various PDE RHS terms (denoted 1d)
  u1_1d   =rep(0,nx); u2_1d =rep(0,nx);u1u2_1d=
     rep(0,nx);
  u1x_1d  =rep(0,nx);u2x_1d =rep(0,nx);
  u1u2x_1d=rep(0,nx);u2xx_1d=rep(0,nx);
```

  Initially, the elements in all of the 1D arrays are zero, and they are then reset (computed) in the subsequent code.

- Similarly, 11 2D arrays are defined via the `matrix` utility (these arrays are identified with `2d` in the names).

```
#
# 2D arrays for plotting (denoted 2d)
  u1x_2d  =matrix(0,nrow=nx,ncol=nout);
  u2x_2d  =matrix(0,nrow=nx,ncol=nout);
  u1u2_2d =matrix(0,nrow=nx,ncol=nout);
  u2xx_2d =matrix(0,nrow=nx,ncol=nout);
  u1u2x_2d=matrix(0,nrow=nx,ncol=nout);
  u1t_2d  =matrix(0,nrow=nx,ncol=nout);
  u2t_2d  =matrix(0,nrow=nx,ncol=nout);
  u1x_2d_anal=matrix(0,nrow=nx,ncol=nout);
  u2x_2d_anal=matrix(0,nrow=nx,ncol=nout);
  u1t_2d_anal=matrix(0,nrow=nx,ncol=nout);
  u2t_2d_anal=matrix(0,nrow=nx,ncol=nout);
```

The column dimension is the number of output points in t, that is, `nout`, which is the length of vector `tout` in Listing 1.1. In this way, the variation of the PDE terms in x and t can be plotted. Initially, all $nx \times nout = 101 \times 6 = 606$ elements in these 2D arrays are zero and then are reset through the subsequent computations.

- The calculations are performed for the six values of t, `t=0,1,2,3,4,5`, with a `for` in `it`. Then, the `n=101` values in x, `x=-10,-9.75,...,15`, are included with a `for` in `ix`.

```
#
# PDE RHS terms
  for(it in 1:nout){
    for(ix in 1:nx){
      u1_1d[ix]=u1_plot[ix,it];
      u2_1d[ix]=u2_plot[ix,it];
    }
```

The numerical solutions computed previously (in Listing 1.1) are placed in two 1D arrays `u1_1d,u2_1d` for the variation of the numerical solutions $u_1(x,t)$ and $u_2(x,t)$ with x (index `ix`).

- First-order derivatives in x are computed by the library differentiator `dss004`.

```
    u1x_1d=dss004(xl,xu,nx,u1_1d);
```

```
u2x_1d=dss004(xl,xu,nx,u2_1d);
u1x_1d[1]=0;u1x_1d[nx]=0;
u2x_1d[1]=0;u2x_1d[nx]=0;
```

where

Derivative	R Variable
$\partial u_1/\partial x$	u1x_1d
$\partial u_2/\partial x$	u2x_1d

BCs (1.4) are then imposed (to correct the boundary derivatives from dss004).

- The nonlinear term and the second derivative in eq. (1.2b) are computed.

```
for(ix in 1:nx){
  u1u2_1d[ix]=u2_1d[ix]/u1_1d[ix]*u1x_1d[ix];
}
u1u2x_1d=dss004(xl,xu,nx,u1u2_1d);
 u2xx_1d=dss004(xl,xu,nx, u2x_1d);
```

where

Derivative	R Variable
$(u_2/u_1)\partial u_1/\partial x$	u1u2_1d
$\partial[(u_2/u_1)\partial u_1/\partial x]/\partial x$	u1u2x_1d
$\partial^2 u_2/\partial x^2$	u2xx_1d

- The 1D terms in x are placed in 2D arrays for subsequent plotting.

```
#
#   2D arrays for plotting
    for(ix in 1:nx){
#
#     Derivatives of solutions in x
#
#     Derivatives of solutions in x
      u1x_2d[ix,it]=u1x_1d[ix];
      u2x_2d[ix,it]=u2x_1d[ix];
      u1u2_2d[ix,it]=u1u2_1d[ix];
      u2xx_2d[ix,it]=u2xx_1d[ix];
      u1u2x_2d[ix,it]=u1u2x_1d[ix];
```

- The derivatives in t according to eqs. (1.2a) and (1.2b) are computed and placed in 2D arrays.

```
#
#     Derivatives of solutions in t
      u1t_2d[ix,it]=-k*u2_1d[ix];
      u2t_2d[ix,it]=D*(u2xx_1d[ix]-2*u1u2x_1d[ix]);
```

where

Derivative	R Variable
$\partial u_1/\partial t$	`u1t_2d`
$\partial u_2/\partial t$	`u2t_2d`

- The analytical derivatives in t are computed by differentiation of eqs. (1.5) with respect to t and placed in 2D arrays.

```
#
#     Analytical derivatives of solutions in t
      expz=exp(-c*(xg[ix]-c*tout[it])/D);
      u1x_2d_anal[ix,it] =(1/c)*(1/(1+expz)^2)*expz*
         (c^2/D);
      u2x_2d_anal[ix,it]=-(1/c)* (c^4/(k*D^2))*expz*
         (1-expz)/(1+expz)^3;
      u1t_2d_anal[ix,it]=-c*u1x_2d_anal[ix,it];
      u2t_2d_anal[ix,it]=-c*u2x_2d_anal[ix,it];
    }
#
# Next t
  }
```

Note the use of the Lagrangian variable $z = x - ct$. The first `}` concludes the `for` in `ix`. The second `}` concludes the `for` in `it`.

- Six terms with 2D arrays are plotted against x with t as a parameter.

$D\partial^2 u_2/\partial x^2$	Fig. 1.3
$-2D\partial[(u_2/u_1)\partial u_1/\partial x]/\partial x$	Fig. 1.4
$\partial u_1/\partial x$	Fig. 1.5
$\partial u_2/\partial x$	Fig. 1.6
$\partial u_1/\partial t$	Fig. 1.7
$\partial u_2/\partial t$	Fig. 1.8

```
#
# Plot Du2_{xx}
  par(mfrow=c(1,1));
  matplot(x=xg,y=D*u2xx_2d,type="l",xlab="x",
    ylab="Du2_{xx}, t=0,1,...,5",xlim=c(xl,xu),
       lty=1,main="Du2_{xx}; t=0,1,...,5;",lwd=2);
                 .            .
                 .            .
                 .            .
    Coding for Figs. (1.4) to (1.8) removed to
       conserve space
                 .            .
                 .            .
                 .            .
#
# End ip = 3
  }
```

The `for` with `ip=3` is then concluded.

We can note the following details about the graphical output.

For Fig. 1.3,

- $D\partial^2 u_2/\partial x^2$ moves left to right as a traveling wave (a function of only $z = x - vt$);
- The form of $D\partial^2 u_2/\partial x^2$ is relatively complex with positive and negative values.

For Fig. 1.4,

- $-2D\partial[(u_2/u1)\partial u_1/\partial x]/\partial x$ moves left to right as a traveling wave (a function of only $z = x - vt$);
- $-2D\partial[(u_2/u_1)\partial u_1/\partial x]/\partial x$ also changes sign as $D\partial^2 u_2/\partial x^2$ of Fig. 1.3. The sum of the terms in Figs. 1.3 and 1.4 produces $\partial u_2/\partial t$ of eq. (1.2b) in a rather complicated way as reflected in Fig. 1.6.

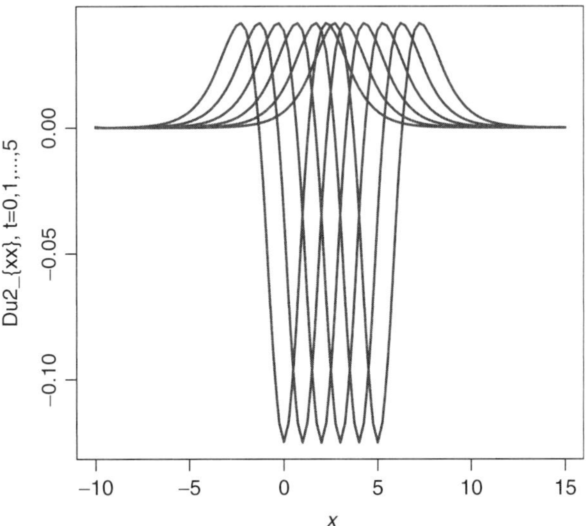

Figure 1.3 $D\partial^2 u_2/\partial x^2$ versus x with t as a parameter.

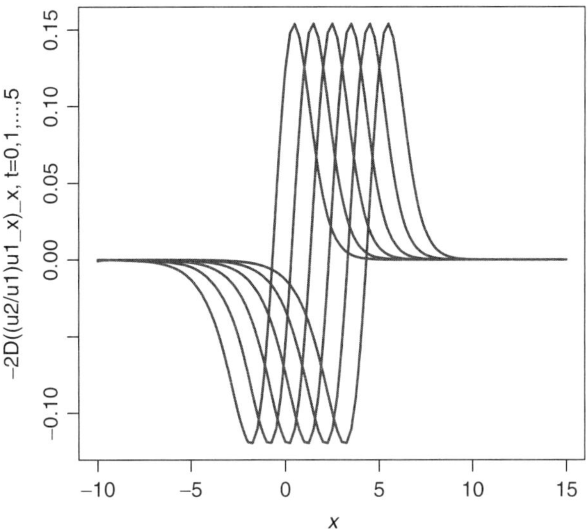

Figure 1.4 $-2D\partial[(u_2/u_1)\partial u_1/\partial x]/\partial x$ versus x with t as a parameter.

For Fig. 1.5,

- $\partial u_1/\partial x$ moves left to right as a traveling wave (a function of only $z = x - vt$);

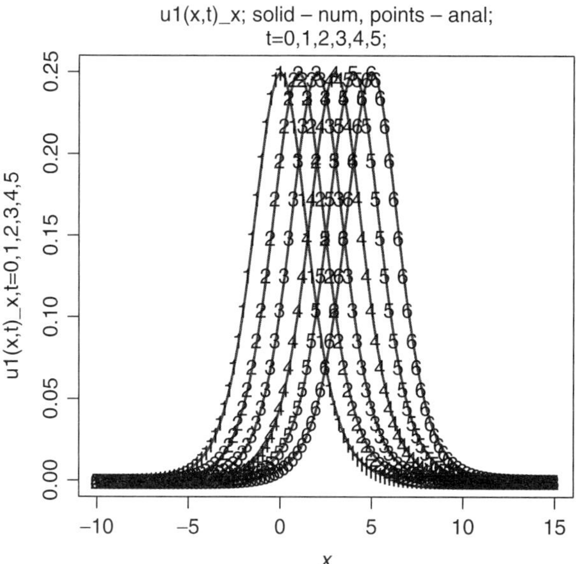

Figure 1.5 $\partial u_1/\partial x$ versus x with t as a parameter.

- The numerical solution $\partial u_1/\partial x \geq 0$, which follows from the calculation by dss004. The analytical $\partial u_1/\partial x \geq 0$ which follows from the analytical solution of eq. (1.5a).
- The solution in Fig. 1.1, $u_1(x, t)$, has only a positive derivative in x as reflected in Fig. 1.5. Also, the location of the largest and smallest values of the derivatives in Fig. 1.5 is reflected in Fig. 1.1.

For Fig. 1.6,

- $\partial u_2/\partial x$ moves left to right as a traveling wave (a function of only $z = x - vt$) and it changes sign;
- The numerical solution $\partial u_2/\partial x$ follows from the calculation by dss004. The analytical solution $\partial u_2/\partial x$ follows from the analytical solution of eq. (1.5b).
- The solution in Fig. 1.2, $u_2(x, t)$, has positive and negative derivatives in x as reflected in Fig. 1.6. In other words, the change in the sign of the derivative in Fig. 1.6 produces a pulse in Fig. 1.2.

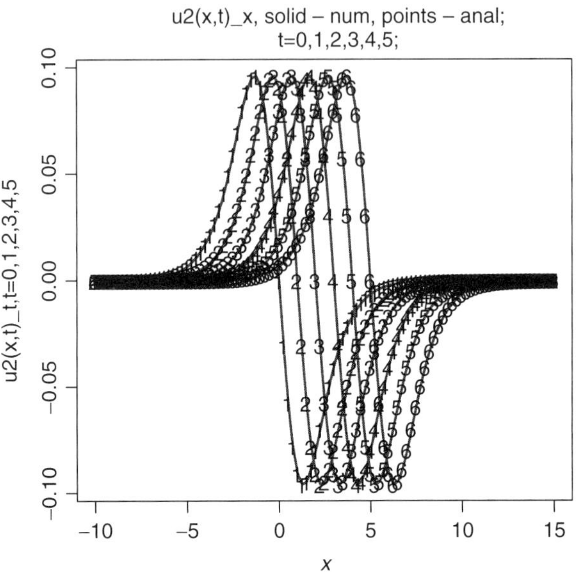

Figure 1.6 $\partial u_2/\partial x$ versus x with t as a parameter.

For Fig. 1.7,

- $\partial u_1/\partial t$ moves left to right as a traveling wave (a function of only $z = x - vt$);
- The numerical solution $\partial u_1/\partial t \leq 0$ follows from the RHS of eq. (1.2a) with $k > 0$. The analytical solution $\partial u_1/\partial t \leq 0$ follows from the analytical solution of eq. (1.5a).

For Fig. 1.8,

- $\partial u_2/\partial t$ moves left to right as a traveling wave (a function of only $z = x - vt$);
- The numerical $\partial u_2/\partial t$ which follows from the RHS of eq. (1.2b). The analytical $\partial u_2/\partial t$ which follows from the analytical solution of eq. (1.5b).

Figures 1.1–1.8 give a detailed explanation of Figs. 1.1 and 1.2. In particular, all of the terms in eqs. (1.2a) and (1.2b) are functions of only $z = x - vt$, that is, $u_1(z)$ and $u_2(z)$, which follows

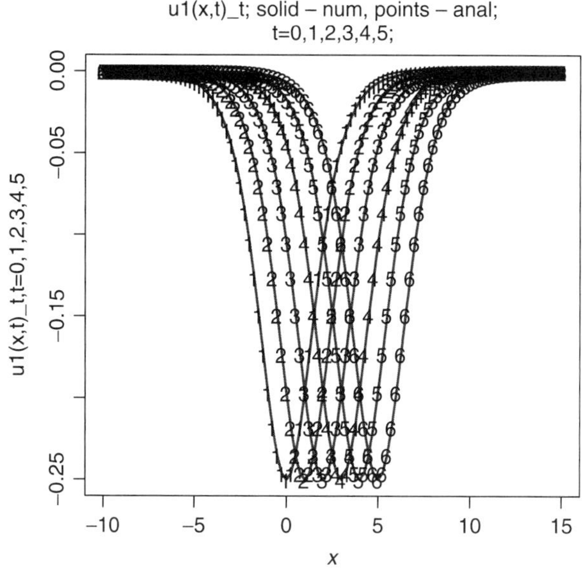

Figure 1.7 $\partial u_1/\partial t$ versus x with t as a parameter.

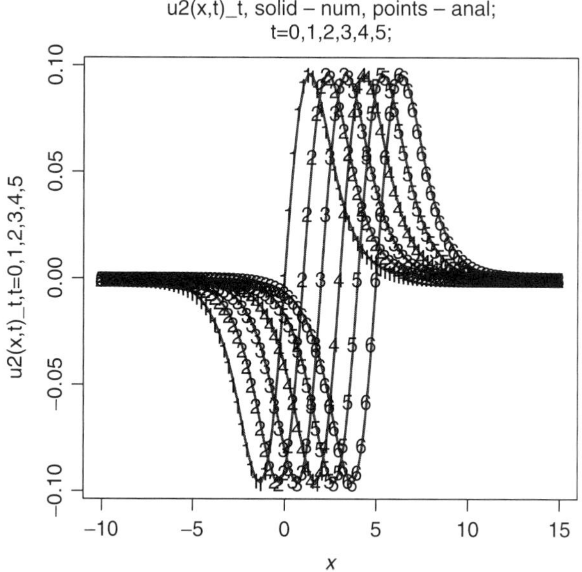

Figure 1.8 $\partial u_2/\partial t$ versus x with t as a parameter.

from eqs. (1.5). And $u_1(x,t)$ and $u_2(x,t) \geq 0$ as required physically because these two dependent variables represent concentrations.

Since the solutions of eqs. (1.5) are functions of z only, we have the following relationships.

$$\frac{\partial u_1}{\partial x} = \frac{du_1}{dz}\frac{\partial z}{\partial x} = \frac{du_1}{dz}(1)$$

$$\frac{\partial u_1}{\partial t} = \frac{du_1}{dz}\frac{\partial z}{\partial t} = \frac{du_1}{dz}(-c)$$

from which it follows that

$$\frac{\partial u_1}{\partial t} = (-c)\frac{\partial u_1}{\partial x} \tag{1.6a}$$

Also, for u_2,

$$\frac{\partial u_2}{\partial t} = (-c)\frac{\partial u_2}{\partial x} \tag{1.6b}$$

Eqs. (1.6) were used previously to compute the analytical $\partial u_1/\partial t, \partial u_2/\partial t$ (in Figs. 1.7 and 1.8) from the analytical solution $\partial u_1/\partial x, \partial u_2/\partial x$ (in Figs. 1.5 and 1.6).

```
u1t_2d_anal[ix,it]=-c*u1x_2d_anal[ix,it];
u2t_2d_anal[ix,it]=-c*u2x_2d_anal[ix,it];
```

(from Listing 1.4). However, the numerical solutions $\partial u_1/\partial x$ and $\partial u_2/\partial x$ were computed by numerical differentiation of the solutions, $u_1(x,t)$ and $u_2(x,t)$ (using dss004), whereas the numerical solutions $\partial u_1/\partial t$ and $\partial u_2/\partial t$ were calculated as the LHS derivatives of eqs. (1.2a) and (1.2b). The agreement of the various derivatives in Figs. 1.5–1.8 illustrates the property that the solutions of eqs. (1.2) are a function of only the Lagrangian variable $z = x - ct$ (a traveling wave solution); this property is stated with eqs. (1.5).

In other words, $\partial u_1/\partial t$ and $\partial u_2/\partial t$ could have been calculated directly from the analytical solutions of eqs. (1.5) (rather than from eqs. (1.6)), but this variation indicates an important property of traveling wave solutions, that is, the partial derivatives in x and t are multiples of $(-c)^{\pm p})$ where p is the order of the derivatives, as illustrated by eq. (1.6) with $p = 1$. The change in the sign of the derivatives in x and t according to eq. (1.6) is evident by comparing Figs. 1.5 and 1.7 and Figs. 1.6 and 1.8.

As a point of terminology, $u_1(x,t), u_2(x,t)$ is termed the Eulerian solution (fixed frame in x), whereas the equivalent $u_1(z), u_2(z)$ is termed the Lagrangian solution (moving frame in x).

1.7 Conclusions

The preceding example of eqs. (1.2) indicates that the calculation of a numerical solution for a nonlinear system of PDEs is straightforward. Further, experimentation with the PDEs can be easily accomplished such as variation of the parameters k, D, c and even the form of the PDEs is straightforward, for example, variation in the RHS of eq. (1.2b).

Additionally, we could drop the nonlinear term in eq. (1.2b), $((u_2/u_1)u_{1x})_x$, and compute a solution to the simplified eq. (1.2b) (now just Fick's second law, eq. (1.1a)). Comparison of the two solutions (with and without $((u_2/u_1)u_{1x})_x$) would give another indication of the effect of this term. For example, eq. (1.1a) would not have a traveling wave solution; rather just conventional diffusion would cause a smoothing of $u_2(x,t)$ to a constant value in x, a fundamentally different type of solution.

In the present example, the analytical solution that could be used to evaluate the accuracy of the numerical solution is available, but this usually is not the case. Rather, we use numerical methods because analytical solutions are generally not available.

The use of library routines such as `lsodes` [3] and `dss004` [1] substantially facilitates the calculation of a numerical PDE solution.

References

[1] Griffiths, G.W. and W.E. Schiesser (2012), *Traveling Wave Analysis of Partial Differential Equations*, Elsevier, Burlington, MA.

[2] Murray, J.D. (2003), *Mathematical Biology, II: Spatial Models and Biomedical Applications*, Third Edition, Springer-Verlag, New York.

[3] Soetaert, K., J. Cash, and F. Mazzia (2012), *Solving Differential Equations in R*, Springer-Verlag, Heidelberg, Germany.

CHAPTER 2

Pattern Formation

2.1 Introduction

The PDE models discussed in this chapter pertain to pattern formation, in this case, a pattern of cells that is defined by a chemoattractant and a stimulant, in analogous manner to the chemotaxis model of Chapter 1. We consider two 1D models based on two PDEs ([2], p 268, eqs. (5.20), (5.21)) and three PDEs ([2], p 264, eqs. (5.11), (5.12), (5.13)). The intent is to demonstrate

- The inclusion of nonlinear terms in the PDEs.
- Adding a PDE to a model that might occur, for example, during model development.
- The calculation and display of the numerical solution of the PDE model, including an examination of the individual terms in the PDEs to provide insight into the origin of the solution properties.

The starting point is the following coupled nonlinear PDE diffusion system ([2], p 264, eqs. (5.11)–(5.13))

$$\frac{\partial u_1}{\partial t} = D_1 \nabla^2 u_1 - \nabla \cdot \left[\frac{k_1 u_1}{(k_2 + u_2)^2} \nabla u_2 \right] + k_3 u_1 \left[\frac{k_4 u_3^2}{k_9 + u_3^2} - u_1 \right] \tag{2.1a}$$

$$\frac{\partial u_2}{\partial t} = D_2 \nabla^2 u_2 + k_5 u_3 \left[\frac{u_1^2}{k_6 + u_1^2} \right] - k_7 u_1 u_2 \tag{2.1b}$$

Differential Equation Analysis in Biomedical Science and Engineering: Partial Differential Equation Applications with R, First Edition. William E. Schiesser.

$$\frac{\partial u_3}{\partial t} = D_3 \nabla^2 u_3 - k_8 u_1 \left[\frac{u_3^2}{k_9 + u_3^2} \right] \tag{2.1c}$$

where

TABLE 2.1 Notation in eqs. (2.1).

Variable	Interpretation
u_1	density of cells
u_2	concentration of chemoattractant
u_3	concentration of stimulant
∇	div operating on a scalar
$\nabla \cdot$	div operating on a vector
$\nabla \cdot \nabla = \nabla^2$	Laplacian
t	time
D_1, D_2, D_3	diffusivities for u_1, u_2, u_3, respectively
$k_1, \ldots, k_9$	rate constants

where $(\cdot)$ denotes a vector dot product.

The ∇ operators in Cartesian coordinates (x, y, z) are given in Table 2.2.

TABLE 2.2 ∇ Operators in Cartesian coordinates.

∇ Operator	Cartesian coordinate representation
∇	$\mathbf{i}\frac{\partial}{\partial x} + \mathbf{j}\frac{\partial}{\partial y} + \mathbf{k}\frac{\partial}{\partial z}$
$\nabla \cdot$	$\left(\mathbf{i}\frac{\partial}{\partial x} + \mathbf{j}\frac{\partial}{\partial y} + \mathbf{k}\frac{\partial}{\partial z}\right) \cdot$
$\nabla \cdot \nabla = \nabla^2$	$\left(\mathbf{i}\frac{\partial}{\partial x} + \mathbf{j}\frac{\partial}{\partial y} + \mathbf{k}\frac{\partial}{\partial z}\right) \cdot \left(\mathbf{i}\frac{\partial}{\partial x} + \mathbf{j}\frac{\partial}{\partial y} + \mathbf{k}\frac{\partial}{\partial z}\right) = \frac{\partial^2}{\partial x^2} + \frac{\partial^2}{\partial y^2} + \frac{\partial^2}{\partial z^2}$

$\mathbf{i}, \mathbf{j}, \mathbf{k}$ are the orthogonal Cartesian unit vectors with the properties, for example, $\mathbf{i} \cdot \mathbf{i} = 1$ and $\mathbf{i} \cdot \mathbf{j} = \mathbf{i} \cdot \mathbf{k} = 0$.

We note that eqs. (2.1) are just three diffusion equations (Fick's second law, $\partial u/\partial t = D\nabla^2 u$) augmented with various nonlinear terms. For example, in eq. (2.1a), $-\nabla \cdot \left[\frac{k_1 u_1}{(k_2+u_2)^2}\nabla u_2\right]$ is a rate of change of the cells (u_1) because of the combined effects of (1) the cells (u_1) from $k_1 u_1$ and (2) the attractant (u_2) from $\frac{1}{(k_2+u_2)^2}\nabla u_2$. The particular form of the nonlinear term, and the numerical values of the parameters, is a matter of experience and judgment employed during the model formulation and most likely will require some trial and error, particularly with regard to reconciliation with experimental data.

Similarly, the nonlinear term $+k_3 u_1\left[\frac{k_4 u_3^2}{k_9+u_3^2} - u_1\right]$ is a rate of change of the cells (u_1) from the combined effects of (1) the cells (u_1) from $+k_3 u_1$ and $-u_1$ (these two terms have opposite signs and therefore opposite effects with $k_3 > 0$) and (2) the stimulant (u_3) from $\frac{k_4 u_3^2}{k_9+u_3^2}$.

In summary, the effect and interaction of these nonlinear terms is complicated. This complexity can be elucidated by computing and examining the individual terms as illustrated in the subsequent programming (for the 3-PDE model).

2.2 Two PDE Model

To start with the 2-PDE model in 1D (x only so that $\nabla^2 = \partial^2/\partial x^2$), dimensionless $u_1(x,t)$ and $u_2(x,t)$ are given by variants of eqs. (2.1a) and (2.1b) ([2], p 268, eqs. (5.20) and (5.21))

$$\frac{\partial u_1}{\partial t} = D_1\frac{\partial^2 u_1}{\partial x^2} - \alpha\frac{\partial}{\partial x}\left[\frac{u_1}{(1+u_2)^2}\frac{\partial u_2}{\partial x}\right] \tag{2.2a}$$

$$\frac{\partial u_2}{\partial t} = \frac{\partial^2 u_2}{\partial x^2} + w\frac{u_1^2}{\mu+u_1^2} \tag{2.2b}$$

where D_1, α, w, and μ are dimensionless constants.

Eqs. (2.2) are first order in t and second order in x. Therefore, each of them requires one IC and two BCs ([1], p 239, eq. (6)).

$$u_1(x,t=0) = f_1(x); \quad u_2(x,t=0) = f_2(x) \tag{2.3a,b}$$

$$\frac{\partial u_1(x=0,t)}{\partial x} = \frac{\partial u_1(x=L,t)}{\partial x} = 0 \tag{2.4a,b}$$

$$\frac{\partial u_2(x=0,t)}{\partial x} = \frac{\partial u_2(x=L,t)}{\partial x} = 0 \tag{2.4c,d}$$

where L is the length of the experimental system. Eqs. (2.4) are zero-flux (no diffusion, homogeneous Neumann) BCs at the physical boundaries of the experimental system.

The nonlinear term in eq. (2.2a) can be expanded as

$$\frac{\partial}{\partial x}\left[\frac{u_1}{(1+u_2)^2}\frac{\partial u_2}{\partial x}\right] = \left[\frac{u_1}{(1+u_2)^2}\frac{\partial^2 u_2}{\partial x^2}\right] + \left[\frac{1}{(1+u_2)^2}\frac{\partial u_1}{\partial x}\frac{\partial u_2}{\partial x}\right] + \left[u_1\frac{-2}{(1+u_2)^3}\left(\frac{\partial u_2}{\partial x}\right)^2\right] \tag{2.5}$$

for use in the subsequent programming.

Eqs. (2.2) to (2.5) constitute the 2-PDE model. We now consider the numerical solution of these equations, starting with the ODE routine based on the MOL.

2.2.1 ODE Routine

The ODE routine with the programming of eqs. (2.2) and (2.5) is in Listing 2.1.

```
  p_form_1=function(t,u,parms){
#
# Function p_form_1 computes the t derivative vector
# of the u1,u2 vectors
#
# One vector to two vectors
  u1=rep(0,nx);u2=rep(0,nx);
  for(i in 1:nx){
    u1[i]=u[i];
    u2[i]=u[i+nx];
  }
#
# u1x, u2x
  u1x=dss004(xl,xu,nx,u1);
```

```
  u2x=dss004(xl,xu,nx,u2);
#
# Boundary conditions
  u1x[1]=0;u1x[nx]=0;
  u2x[1]=0;u2x[nx]=0;
  nl=2;nu=2;
#
# u1xx, u2xx
  u1xx=dss044(xl,xu,nx,u1,u1x,nl,nu);
  u2xx=dss044(xl,xu,nx,u2,u2x,nl,nu);
#
# RHS terms
  term1=rep(0,nx);term2=rep(0,nx);term3=rep(0,nx);
  for(i in 1:nx){
    den=1/(1+u2[i])^2;
    term1[i]=u1[i]*den*u2xx[i];
    term2[i]=den*u1x[i]*u2x[i];
    term3[i]=-2*u1[i]*den/(1+u2[i])*u2x[i]^2;
  }
#
# PDEs
  u1t=rep(0,nx);u2t=rep(0,nx);
  for(i in 1:nx){
    u1t[i]=d1*u1xx[i]-alpha*(term1[i]+term2[i]+term3[i]);
    u2t[i]=u2xx[i]+w1*u1[i]^2/(mu+u1[i]^2);
  }
#
# Two vectors to one vector
  ut=rep(0,2*nx);
  for(i in 1:nx){
    ut[i]    =u1t[i];
    ut[i+nx]=u2t[i];
  }
#
# Increment calls to p_form_1
  ncall <<- ncall+1;
#
# Return derivative vector
  return(list(c(ut)));
}
```

Listing 2.1 ODE routine `p_form_1`.

We can note the following details about p_form_1.

- The function is defined.

```
  p_form_1=function(t,u,parms){
#
# Function p_form_1 computes the t derivative vector
# of the u1,u2 vectors
```

  The input arguments are in conformity with the R ODE integrators, in this case lsodes called by the main program discussed subsequently. lsodes in turn calls p_form_1. u is a vector of 102 elements, that is, 51 points in x for each of eqs. (2.2) (102 ODEs in the MOL approximation of eqs. (2.2)). parms is unused.

- u is placed in two vectors, u1 and u2, to facilitate subsequent programming in terms of problem-oriented variables, that is, the dependent variables of eqs. (2.2). nx=51 is set in the main program.

```
#
# One vector to two vectors
  u1=rep(0,nx);u2=rep(0,nx);
  for(i in 1:nx){
    u1[i]=u[i];
    u2[i]=u[i+nx];
  }
```

- $\partial u_1/\partial x, \partial u_2/\partial x$ are computed by the library differentiator dss004. xl and xu are set in the main program.

```
#
# u1x, u2x
  u1x=dss004(xl,xu,nx,u1);
  u2x=dss004(xl,xu,nx,u2);
```

- BCs (2.4) are programmed.

```
#
# Boundary conditions
  u1x[1]=0;u1x[nx]=0;
```

```
  u2x[1]=0;u2x[nx]=0;
  nl=2;nu=2;
```

Since the BCs specify the partial derivatives at the boundaries, that is, $\partial u_1(x=0,t)/\partial x = 0$, $\partial u_1(x=L,t)/\partial x = 0$, and similar conditions for u_2, Neumann BCs are designated with `nl` and `nu`.

- $\partial^2 u_1/\partial x^2$ and $\partial^2 u_2/\partial x^2$ are computed by the library differentiator `dss044`.

```
#
# u1xx, u2xx
  u1xx=dss044(xl,xu,nx,u1,u1x,nl,nu);
  u2xx=dss044(xl,xu,nx,u2,u2x,nl,nu);
```

Note that the derivatives at the boundaries, `u1x[1],u1x[nx]` and `u2x[1],u2x[nx]`, are inputs to `dss044`.

- The programming of the three RHS terms in eq. (2.5) is programmed with a `for` with index `i`.

```
#
# RHS terms
  term1=rep(0,nx);term2=rep(0,nx);term3=rep(0,nx);
  for(i in 1:nx){
    den=1/(1+u2[i])^2;
    term1[i]=u1[i]*den*u2xx[i];
    term2[i]=den*u1x[i]*u2x[i];
    term3[i]=-2*u1[i]*den/(1+u2[i])*u2x[i]^2;
  }
```

The correspondence between the terms in eq. (2.5) and their coding is

$$\frac{1}{(1+u_2)^2} \Rightarrow$$

```
den=1/(1+u2[i])^2;
```

$$\left[\frac{u_1}{(1+u_2)^2}\frac{\partial^2 u_2}{\partial x^2}\right] \Rightarrow$$

```
term1[i]=u1[i]*den*u2xx[i];
```

$$\left[\frac{1}{(1+u_2)^2}\frac{\partial u_1}{\partial x}\frac{\partial u_2}{\partial x}\right] \Rightarrow$$

```
term2[i]=den*u1x[i]*u2x[i];
```

$$\left[u_1\frac{-2}{(1+u_2)^3}\left(\frac{\partial u_2}{\partial x}\right)^2\right] \Rightarrow$$

```
term3[i]=-2*u1[i]*den/(1+u2[i])*u2x[i]^2;
```

- Eqs. (2.2) are programmed in a `for` with index `i`.

```
#
# PDEs
  u1t=rep(0,nx);u2t=rep(0,nx);
  for(i in 1:nx){
    u1t[i]=d1*u1xx[i]-alpha*(term1[i]+term2[i]
       +term3[i]);
    u2t[i]=u2xx[i]+w1*u1[i]^2/(mu+u1[i]^2);
  }
```

`d1,alpha,w1,mu` are defined numerically in the main program. The derivatives $\partial u_1/\partial t, \partial u_2/\partial t$ in `u1t,u2t` are the final result. They are passed to `lsodes` for the integration of the `102` ODEs.

- The derivatives `u1t,u2t` are placed in a single vector `ut` that is returned to `lsodes` for the integration of the `102` ODEs.

```
#
# Two vectors to one vector
  ut=rep(0,2*nx);
  for(i in 1:nx){
    ut[i]   =u1t[i];
    ut[i+nx]=u2t[i];
  }
```

- The number of calls to `p_form_1` is incremented, and the value is returned to the main program with `<<-`. The derivative vector is then returned from p_form_1 as a list (as required by the R ODE integrators including lsodes).

```
#
# Increment calls to p_form_1
  ncall <<- ncall+1;
#
# Return derivative vector
  return(list(c(ut)));
}
```

The final } concludes p_form_1.

In summary, the model consisting of eqs. (2.2), (2.4), and (2.5) is programmed in p_form_1. The only part of the model not included in this routine are the ICs for eqs. (2.2), that is, eqs. (2.3), to start the numerical solution. We now consider the effect of different ICs and some features of the numerical and graphical outputs produced by the main program.

2.2.2 Main Program

p_form_1 is called by the main program in Listing 2.2 as an input argument of lsodes.

```
#
# Access ODE integrator
  library("deSolve");
#
# Access functions for numerical  solutions
  setwd("c:/R/bme_pde/chap2/v_2pde");
  source("p_form_1.R");
  source("dss004.R");
  source("dss044.R");
#
# Level of output
#
#   ip = 1 - graphical (plotted) solutions
#            (u1(x,t), u2(x,t)) only
#
```

```
#   ip = 2 - numerical and graphical solutions
#
  ip=2;
#
# Initial condition (IC)
#
#   ncase = 1 - spatially uniform
#
#   ncase = 2 - Gaussian
#
#   ncase = 3 - step
#
  ncase=1;
#
# Grid (in x)
  nx=51;xl=0;xu=1;
  xg=seq(from=xl,to=xu,by=0.02);
#
# Parameters
  alpha=10;d1=0.5;w1=1;mu=0.1;
  cat(sprintf(
    "\n\n  alpha = %5.2f  d1 = %5.2f   w1 = %5.2f
       mu = %5.2f\n",alpha,d1,w1,mu));
#
# Independent variable for ODE integration
  nout=11;
  tout=seq(from=0,to=0.25,by=0.025);
#
# Initial condition
  u0=rep(0,2*nx);u10=rep(0,nx);u20=rep(0,nx);
  for(i in 1:nx){
#
#   Solution remains spatially uniform
    if(ncase==1){
    u10[i]=1;u20[i]=0;}
#
#   Initial Gaussian in u1
    if(ncase==2){
    u10[i]=exp(-5*(xg[i]-0.5)^2);u20[i]=0;}
#
#   Initial band in u1
```

```
    if(ncase==3){
    if(i<=11){
      u10[i]=1;u20[i]=0;
    }else{
      u10[i]=0;u20[i]=0;
    } }
    u0[i]   =u10[i];
    u0[i+nx]=u20[i];
  }
  t=0;
  ncall=0;
#
# ODE integration
  out=lsodes(y=u0,times=tout,func=p_form_1,parms=NULL)
  nrow(out)
  ncol(out)
#
# Arrays for plotting numerical solution
  u1_plot=matrix(0,nrow=nx,ncol=nout);
  u2_plot=matrix(0,nrow=nx,ncol=nout);
  for(it in 1:nout){
    for(ix in 1:nx){
       u1_plot[ix,it]=out[it,ix+1];
       u2_plot[ix,it]=out[it,ix+1+nx];
    }
  }
#
# Display numerical solution
  if(ip==2){
    for(it in 1:nout){
     cat(sprintf("\n   t    x   u1(x,t)  u2(x,t)\n"));
      for(ix in 1:nx){
        cat(sprintf("%7.3f%8.2f%12.5f%12.5f\n",
        tout[it],xg[ix],u1_plot[ix,it],u2_plot[ix,it]));
      }
    }
  }
#
# Calls to ODE routine
  cat(sprintf("\n\n ncall = %5d\n\n",ncall));
#
```

```
# Plot u1 numerical
  par(mfrow=c(1,1));
  matplot(x=xg,y=u1_plot,type="l",xlab="x",
          ylab="u1(x,t), t=0,0.025,...,0.25",xlim=c
             (xl,xu),lty=1,main="u1(x,t); t=0,0.025,...,
                0.25;",lwd=2);
#
# Plot u2 numerical
  par(mfrow=c(1,1));
  matplot(x=xg,y=u2_plot,type="l",xlab="x",
          ylab="u2(x,t), t=0,0.025,...,0.25",xlim=c
             (xl,xu),lty=1,main="u2(x,t); t=0,0.025,...,
                0.25;",lwd=2);
```

Listing 2.2 Main program for eqs. (2.2).

We can note the following details about this main program.

- The R ODE integrator library, `deSolve`, is accessed to provide `lsodes`. `p_form_1` of Listing 2.1 and the two spatial differentiation routines used in `p_form_1` are accessed by `setwd` (set working directory) and `source` statements.

```
#
# Access ODE integrator
  library("deSolve");
#
# Access functions for numerical solutions
  setwd("c:/R/bme_pde/chap2/v_2pde");
  source("p_form_1.R");
  source("dss004.R");
  source("dss044.R");
```

  Note the use of the forward slash / in the `setwd`.

- The level of output is specified with `ip`.

```
#
# Level of output
#
```

```
#    ip = 1 - graphical (plotted) solutions
#             (u1(x,t), u2(x,t)) only
#
#    ip = 2 - numerical and graphical solutions
#
  ip=2;
```

- One of the three ICs is selected with ncase. The details of each IC will be clear from the subsequent programming.

```
#
# Initial condition (IC)
#
#    ncase = 1 - spatially uniform
#
#    ncase = 2 - Gaussian
#
#    ncase = 3 - step
#
  ncase=1;
```

- The grid in x is defined as $0 \leq x \leq 1$, with 51 points so that $x = 0, 0.02, \ldots, 1$.

```
#
# Grid (in x)
  nx=51;xl=0;xu=1;
  xg=seq(from=xl,to=xu,by=0.02);
```

- The parameters of eqs. (2.2) are assigned numerical values as suggested in [2], p269 and then displayed at the beginning of the solution.

```
#
# Parameters
  alpha=10;d1=0.5;w1=1;mu=0.1;
  cat(sprintf(
   "\n\n  alpha = %5.2f   d1 = %5.2f    w1 = %5.2f
      mu = %5.2f\n",alpha,d1,w1,mu));
```

- The interval in t is $0 \leq t \leq 0.25$ with 11 values, $t = 0, 0.025, \ldots, 0.25$, for the output.

```
#
# Independent variable for ODE integration
  nout=11;
  tout=seq(from=0,to=0.25,by=0.025);
```

- Three ICs are programmed.

ncase=1, $u_1(x, t = 0) = 1, u_2(x, t = 0) = 0.$

ncase=2, $u_1(x, t = 0) =$ gaussian function, $u_2(x, t = 0) = 0.$

ncase=3, $u_1(x, t = 0) = 1, u_2(x, t = 0) = 0,\ 0 \leq x \leq 0.025,$

$u_1(x, t = 0) = 0, u_2(x, t = 0) = 0,\ 0.025 < x \leq 0.25.$

```
#
# Initial condition
  u0=rep(0,2*nx);u10=rep(0,nx);u20=rep(0,nx);
  for(i in 1:nx){
#
#   Solution remains spatially uniform
    if(ncase==1){
    u10[i]=1;u20[i]=0;}
#
#   Initial Gaussian in u1
    if(ncase==2){
    u10[i]=exp(-5*(xg[i]-0.5)^2);u20[i]=0;}
#
#   Initial band in u1
    if(ncase==3){
    if(i<=11){
      u10[i]=1;u20[i]=0;
    }else{
      u10[i]=0;u20[i]=0;
    } }
    u0[i]   =u10[i];
    u0[i+nx]=u20[i];
  }
  t=0;
  ncall=0;
```

The ICs, u10,u20, are then placed in a single vector, u0, of length $2(51) = 102$. Finally, the independent variable t and the number of calls to p_form_1 are initialized.

- The ODEs are integrated by lsodes, which is informed of the number of ODEs (102) by the length of the IC vector u0.

```
#
# ODE integration
  out=lsodes(y=u0,times=tout,func=p_form_1,
     parms=NULL)
  nrow(out)
  ncol(out)
```

Note the use of the IC vector, u0, the vector of output points, tout, and the ODE routine p_form_1 of Listing 2.1. y,times,func,parms are reserved names. parms is unused. The dimensions of the solution array, out, are displayed for verification.

- The solution is put into two 2D arrays, u1_plot,u2_plot, for subsequent plotting.

```
#
# Arrays for plotting numerical solution
  u1_plot=matrix(0,nrow=nx,ncol=nout);
  u2_plot=matrix(0,nrow=nx,ncol=nout);
  for(it in 1:nout){
    for(ix in 1:nx){
       u1_plot[ix,it]=out[it,ix+1];
       u2_plot[ix,it]=out[it,ix+1+nx];
    }
  }
```

Note the offset of 1 in the second subscript of out, e.g., ix+1, since the values of t are included in out as out[it,1] (this is the usual operation of lsodes and the other R ODE integrators). In other words, out has the dimensions out[nout,2*nx+1]=out[6,2*51+1]=out[6,103].

- For ip=2, the numerical solution is displayed in tabular form.

```
#
# Display numerical solution
  if(ip==2){
    for(it in 1:nout){
      cat(sprintf("\n     t     x      u1(x,t)
         u2(x,t)\n"));
      for(ix in 1:nx){
        cat(sprintf("%7.3f%8.2f%12.5f%12.5f\n",
        tout[it],xg[ix],u1_plot[ix,it],u2_plot
           [ix,it]));
      }
    }
  }
```

- The number of calls to `p_form_1` is displayed at the end of the solution as a measure of the computational effort to compute the solution.

```
#
# Calls to ODE routine
  cat(sprintf("\n\n ncall = %5d\n\n",ncall));
```

- $u_1(x,t), u_2(x,t)$ are plotted as a function of x with t as a parameter.

```
#
# Plot u1 numerical
  par(mfrow=c(1,1));
  matplot(x=xg,y=u1_plot,type="l",xlab="x",
         ylab="u1(x,t), t=0,0.025,...,0.25",xlim=c
            (xl,xu),lty=1,main="u1(x,t); t=0,0.025,...,
               0.25;",lwd=2);
#
# Plot u2 numerical
  par(mfrow=c(1,1));
  matplot(x=xg,y=u2_plot,type="l",xlab="x",
         ylab="u2(x,t), t=0,0.025,...,0.25",xlim=c
            (xl,xu),lty=1,main="u2(x,t); t=0,0.025,...,
               0.25;",lwd=2);
```

`par(mfrow=c(1,1))` specifies a 1×1 matrix of plots, that is, a single plot. `matplot` produces the parametric plots by using `xg` as the abscissa (horizontal, x variable) and u1_plot,u2_plot as the ordinate (vertical, y variable), with the requirement that the number of rows of x and y must be the same, in this case 51.

This concludes the programming of eqs. (2.2) to (2.5). The numerical and graphical outputs are reviewed in the following sections.

2.2.3 Numerical Solution

For ncase=1, abbreviated numerical output (from ip=2 in Listing 2.2) is listed in Table 2.3.

We can note the following details about this output.

- The dimensions of out are out[11,103] as expected (and explained previously).
- The ICs, $u_1(x,t=0)=1, u_2(x,t=0)=0$ for ncase=1, are correct (always a good idea to check the ICs so the solution starts correctly).

TABLE 2.3 Abbreviated output from Listing 2.2 with ip=2 for ncase=1.

```
alpha = 10.00  d1 =  0.50   w1 =  1.00  mu =  0.10

> nrow(out)
[1] 11
> ncol(out)
[1] 103

     t        x      u1(x,t)      u2(x,t)
 0.000     0.00      1.00000      0.00000
 0.000     0.02      1.00000      0.00000
 0.000     0.04      1.00000      0.00000
 0.000     0.06      1.00000      0.00000
 0.000     0.08      1.00000      0.00000
 0.000     0.10      1.00000      0.00000
             .         .
             .         .
             .         .
```

(*continued*)

TABLE 2.3 (*Continued*)

```
 Output for x = 0.12 to 0.88 removed
           .        .
           .        .
           .        .
0.000    0.90     1.00000     0.00000
0.000    0.92     1.00000     0.00000
0.000    0.94     1.00000     0.00000
0.000    0.96     1.00000     0.00000
0.000    0.98     1.00000     0.00000
0.000    1.00     1.00000     0.00000
           .        .
           .        .
           .        .
 Output for t = 0.025 to 0.225 removed
           .        .
           .        .
           .        .
    t       x     u1(x,t)     u2(x,t)
0.250    0.00     1.00000     0.22727
0.250    0.02     1.00000     0.22727
0.250    0.04     1.00000     0.22727
0.250    0.06     1.00000     0.22727
0.250    0.08     1.00000     0.22727
0.250    0.10     1.00000     0.22727
           .        .
           .        .
           .        .
 Output for x = 0.12 to 0.88 removed
           .        .
           .        .
           .        .
0.250    0.90     1.00000     0.22727
0.250    0.92     1.00000     0.22727
0.250    0.94     1.00000     0.22727
0.250    0.96     1.00000     0.22727
0.250    0.98     1.00000     0.22727
0.250    1.00     1.00000     0.22727
```

TABLE 2.3 (*Continued*)

```
ncall =   129

Warning message:
In plot.window(...) :
relative range of values =  27 * EPS, is small (axis 2)
```

- The solutions, $u_1(x,t), u_2(x,t)$, remain invariant with x to six figures. This result follows from eqs. (2.2). For the ICs that are invariant with x, $\partial u_1(x,t=0)/\partial x = \partial u_2(x,t=0)/\partial x = 0$. Thus, the zero derivatives in x in eq (2.2a) lead to $\partial u_1(x,t)/\partial t = 0$ for all x, that is, $u_1(x,t)$ is invariant in t so that $u_1(x,t=0) = u_1(x,t) = 1$ for all t as well as x as observed in Table 2.3.

  For eq. (2.2b), the zero derivative in x gives the PDE $\dfrac{\partial u_2}{\partial t} = w\dfrac{u_1^2}{\mu + u_1^2}$. With $w = 1$, $\mu = 0.1$ (from Listing 2.2), $\dfrac{\partial u_2}{\partial t} = (1)1^2/(0.1 + 1^2) = 1/1.1 = 0.9090\ldots$. In other words, $u_2(x,t)$ changes by $0.9090\ldots$ for each unit change in t. For a change in t from 0 to 0.250 (in Table 2.3), the change in u_2 from 0 is $(0.9090\ldots)(0.25) = 0.227272\ldots$ as indicated in Table 2.3.
- The computational effort is modest with `ncall = 129`.
- Unexpectedly, the `matplot` utility applied to u_1 could not automatically scale the constant $u_1(x,t) = 1.00000$ solution vertically and therefore issued an error message.

  ```
  Warning message:
  In plot.window(...) :
  relative range of values =  27 * EPS, is small
     (axis 2)
  ```

  The resulting plot is in Fig. 2.1. Various attempts to rescale $u_1(x,t)$ so that `matplot` would produce a satisfactory plot (rather than Fig. 2.1), including the use of the argument `ylim` for `matplot` (forced rather than automatic scaling), were unsuccessful (perhaps the reader would like to retry some rescaling of $u_1(x,t)$). Interestingly, `matplot` had no difficulty in plotting $u_2(x,t)$ as indicated in Fig. 2.2.

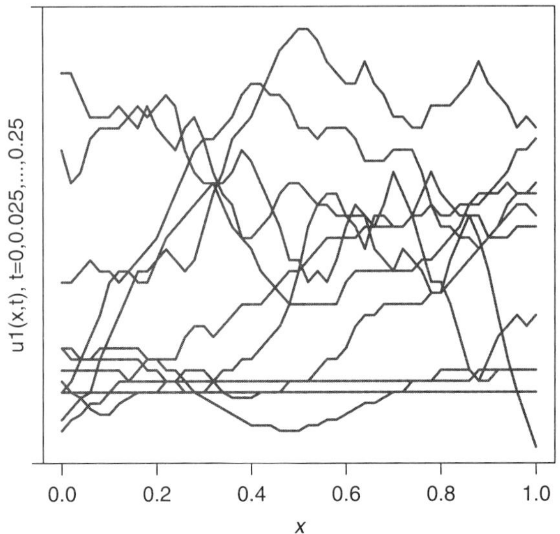

Figure 2.1 $u_1(x,t)$ versus x with t as a parameter, `ncase=1`.

Fig. 2.2 indicates the constant $u_2(x,t)$ in x of Table 2.3, with the variation of $0.9090\ldots$ for each unit in t as discussed previously.

For `ncase=2`, the abbreviated numerical output (from `ip=2` in Listing 2.2) is listed in Table 2.4.

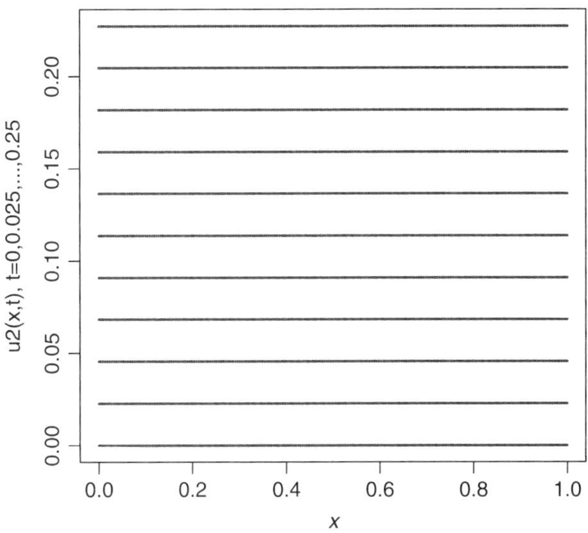

Figure 2.2 $u_2(x,t)$ versus x with t as a parameter, `ncase=1`.

TABLE 2.4 Abbreviated output from Listing 2.2 with `ip=2` for `ncase=2`.

```
alpha = 10.00  d1 =  0.50   w1 =  1.00  mu =  0.10

> nrow(out)
[1] 11
> ncol(out)
[1] 103

     t        x      u1(x,t)      u2(x,t)
 0.000     0.00      0.28650      0.00000
 0.000     0.02      0.31600      0.00000
 0.000     0.04      0.34715      0.00000
 0.000     0.06      0.37984      0.00000
 0.000     0.08      0.41395      0.00000
 0.000     0.10      0.44933      0.00000
              .        .
              .        .
              .        .
  Output for x = 0.12 to 0.88 removed
              .        .
              .        .
              .        .
 0.000     0.90      0.44933      0.00000
 0.000     0.92      0.41395      0.00000
 0.000     0.94      0.37984      0.00000
 0.000     0.96      0.34715      0.00000
 0.000     0.98      0.31600      0.00000
 0.000     1.00      0.28650      0.00000
              .        .
              .        .
              .        .
  Output for t = 0.025 to 0.225 removed
              .        .
              .        .
              .        .
     t        x      u1(x,t)      u2(x,t)
 0.250     0.00      0.69716      0.20672
 0.250     0.02      0.69720      0.20673
```

(continued)

TABLE 2.4 (*Continued*)

```
0.250     0.04      0.69732      0.20673
0.250     0.06      0.69753      0.20673
0.250     0.08      0.69781      0.20674
0.250     0.10      0.69816      0.20674
             .         .
             .         .
             .         .
 Output for x = 0.12 to 0.88 removed
             .         .
             .         .
             .         .
0.250     0.90      0.69816      0.20674
0.250     0.92      0.69781      0.20674
0.250     0.94      0.69753      0.20673
0.250     0.96      0.69732      0.20673
0.250     0.98      0.69720      0.20673

ncall =    258
```

We can note the following details about this output.

- The ICs, $u_1(x, t = 0)$ = gaussian function, $u_2(x, t = 0) = 0$ for `ncase=2`, appear to be correct, including symmetry around $x = 0.5$ for $u_1(x, t = 0)$ (v. the Gaussian IC function programmed in Listing 2.2 to explain this symmetry); the numbers for $u_1(x, t = 0)$ can be easily checked.
- $u_1(x, t)$ varies with x (starting at $t = 0$) so that the x derivatives in eq. (2.2a) also vary with x (and are therefore nonzero). Thus, $\partial u_1/\partial t$ from eq. (2.2a) now changes with x and t as reflected in Table 2.4. For eq. (2.2b), the coupling between eqs. (2.2a) and (2.2b), and the nonzero derivative in x, gives the PDE $\frac{\partial u_2}{\partial t}$ a variation in x and t.
- The computational effort is modest with `ncall = 258`.
- The plots of $u_1(x, t)$ and $u_2(x, t)$ in Figs. 2.3 and 2.4 give a more complete picture than the abbreviated output in Table 2.4. $u_1(x, t)$ has the pronounced Gaussian function at $t = 0$ (the

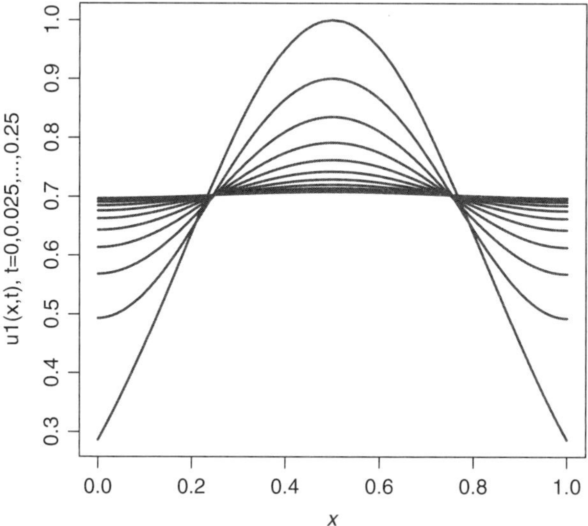

Figure 2.3 $u_1(x,t)$ versus x with t as a parameter, `ncase=2`.

IC for eq. (2.2a)). Through the effect of diffusion (expressed through the derivatives in x), $u_1(x,t)$ moves toward a uniform value with increasing t. Note the discontinuity between the IC (Gaussian function) at $x = 0, L$ and the BCs (eqs. (2.4)).

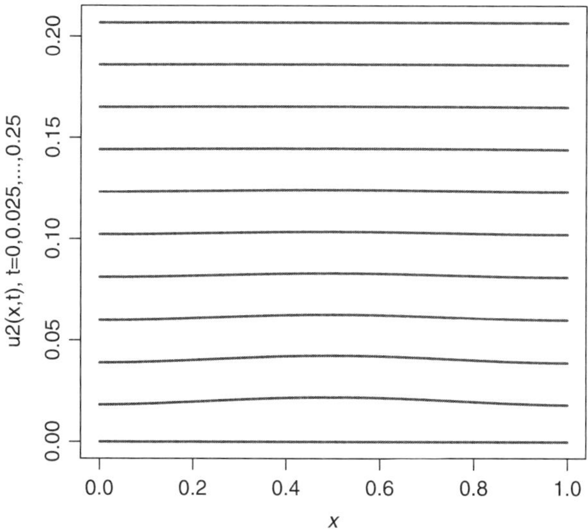

Figure 2.4 $u_2(x,t)$ versus x with t as a parameter, `ncase=2`.

At $t = 0$, the derivatives from the IC, $\partial u_1(x = 0, t = 0)/\partial x$ and $\partial u_1(x = L, t = 0)/\partial x$, are not zero (from the Gaussian function), whereas they are zero from BCs (eqs. 2.4). This discontinuity could be accommodated numerically because of the smoothing effect of the diffusion (expressed through the derivatives in x). This smoothing is a general property of parabolic PDEs.
The variation of $u_2(x,t)$ with x is small, and for increasing t, this variation essentially approaches zero as reflected in Table 2.4 (e.g., at $t = 0.250$).

For `ncase=3`, the abbreviated numerical output (from `ip=2` in Listing 2.2) is listed in Table 2.5.

We can note the following details about this output.

- The ICs, $u_1(x, t = 0) =$ unit step at $x = 0.025$, $u_2(x, t = 0) = 0$ for `ncase=3`, appear to be correct (the ICs at $t = 0$ are abbreviated to conserve space).
- $u_1(x,t)$ varies with x (starting as a unit step at $t = 0$) so that the x derivatives in eq. (2.2a) also vary with x (and are therefore nonzero). Thus, $\partial u_1/\partial t$ from eq. (2.2a) now changes with x and t as reflected in Table 2.5. For eq. (2.2b), the coupling between eqs. (2.2a) and (2.2b) and the nonzero derivative in x give the PDE $\dfrac{\partial u_2}{\partial t}$ a variation in x and t.
- The computational effort is modest with `ncall = 302`.
- The plots of $u_1(x,t)$ and $u_2(x,t)$ in Figs. 2.5 and 2.6 give a more complete picture than the abbreviated output in Table 2.5. $u_1(x,t)$ is the unit step at $t = 0$ (the IC for eq. (2.2a)). Through the effect of diffusion (expressed through the derivatives in x), $u_1(x,t)$ moves toward a uniform value with increasing t. The fact that this discontinuity could be accommodated numerically is due to the smoothing effect of the diffusion, a property of parabolic PDEs.
Also, the IC (unit step) and the BCs are consistent at $x = 0, L$ (the derivatives in x from the IC and BCs (2.4) are zero, that is, $\partial u_1(x = 0, t = 0)/\partial x = \partial u_1(x = L, t = 0)/\partial x = 0$).

TABLE 2.5 Abbreviated output from Listing 2.2 with `ip=2` for `ncase=3`.

```
alpha = 10.00  d1 =  0.50   w1 =  1.00  mu =  0.10

> nrow(out)
[1] 11
> ncol(out)
[1] 103

     t        x      u1(x,t)      u2(x,t)
 0.000     0.00      1.00000      0.00000
 0.000     0.02      1.00000      0.00000
 0.000     0.04      1.00000      0.00000
 0.000     0.06      1.00000      0.00000
 0.000     0.08      1.00000      0.00000
 0.000     0.10      1.00000      0.00000
              .        .
              .        .
              .        .
  Output for x = 0.12 to 0.88 removed
              .        .
              .        .
              .        .
 0.000     0.90      0.00000      0.00000
 0.000     0.92      0.00000      0.00000
 0.000     0.94      0.00000      0.00000
 0.000     0.96      0.00000      0.00000
 0.000     0.98      0.00000      0.00000
 0.000     1.00      0.00000      0.00000
              .        .
              .        .
              .        .
  Output for t = 0.025 to 0.225 removed
              .        .
              .        .
              .        .
     t        x      u1(x,t)      u2(x,t)
 0.250     0.00      0.43586      0.10479
```

(*continued*)

TABLE 2.5 *(Continued)*

```
 0.250     0.02      0.43513      0.10471
 0.250     0.04      0.43295      0.10449
 0.250     0.06      0.42935      0.10412
 0.250     0.08      0.42436      0.10360
 0.250     0.10      0.41806      0.10294
            .         .
            .         .
            .         .
  Output for x = 0.12 to 0.88 removed
            .         .
            .         .
            .         .
 0.250     0.90      0.05976      0.03969
 0.250     0.92      0.05834      0.03921
 0.250     0.94      0.05724      0.03885
 0.250     0.96      0.05646      0.03858
 0.250     0.98      0.05599      0.03843
 0.250     1.00      0.05584      0.03837

 ncall =   302
```

The smoothing of the unit step at $x = 0.025$ is clear in Figs. 2.5 and 2.6.

In conclusion, the interaction between eqs. (2.2a) and (2.2b) is rather complicated but can be studied numerically and graphically through experimentation with the R routines in Listings 2.1 and 2.2. For example, the three ICs for `ncase=1,2,3` could be easily studied. The same is true for variations in the PDE parameters and even for the number and form (structure) of the PDEs. This is demonstrated next where the number of PDEs is increased from two to three.

Also, the question of the accuracy of the numerical solutions was not addressed. To address this, the number of grid points in x could be changed (from 51) and the effect on the solutions observed, an application of h refinement. Similarly, the order of the spatial differentiators (e.g., `dss004,dss044`) could be changed (e.g., by calling

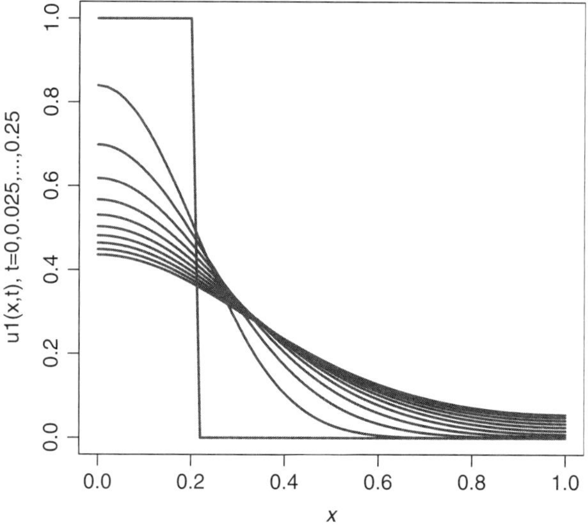

Figure 2.5 $u_1(x,t)$ versus x with t as a parameter, `ncase=3`.

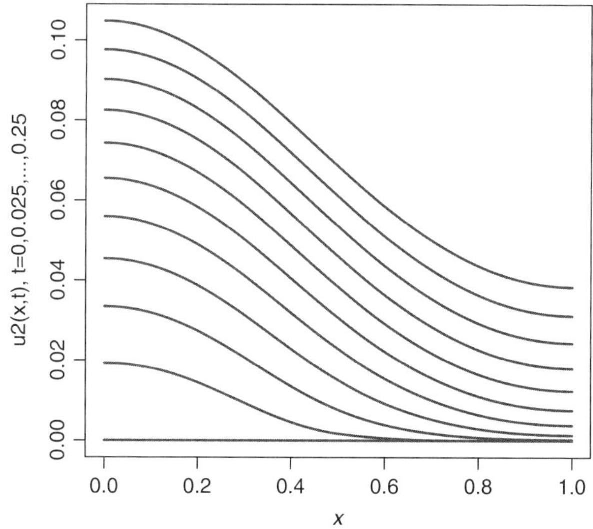

Figure 2.6 $u_2(x,t)$ versus x with t as a parameter, `ncase=3`.

routines with different orders in `p_form_1`), a form of p refinement. This form of error analysis should be a standard procedure for new PDE applications and is demonstrated in the analysis of the 3-PDE model that follows.

2.3 Three PDE Model

The model of eqs. (2.2) to (2.5) is now extended by adding a PDE for the stimulant Also, dimensional variables will be used rather than the dimensionless variables of eqs. (2.2) to (2.5). The resulting 3-PDE model follows ([2], p 264).

$$\frac{\partial u_1}{\partial t} = D_1 \nabla^2 u_1 - \nabla\left[\frac{k_1 u_1}{(k_2+u_2)^2}\nabla u_2\right] + k_3 u_1\left(\frac{k_4 u_3^2}{k_9+u_3^2} - u_1\right) \tag{2.6a}$$

$$\frac{\partial u_2}{\partial t} = D_2 \nabla^2 u_2 + k_5 u_3\left(\frac{u_1^2}{k_6+u_1^2} - k_7 u_1 u_2\right) \tag{2.6b}$$

$$\frac{\partial u_3}{\partial t} = D_3 \nabla^2 u_3 - k_8 u_1\left(\frac{u_3^2}{k_9+u_3^2}\right) \tag{2.6c}$$

where u_3 is the stimulant concentration.

The parameters of eqs. (2.6) with numerical values and units are listed in Table (2.6 [2], p 266, Table 5.1). Five parameters, u_{20}, k_5, k_6, k_7, and k_8, are not given by Murray and therefore are estimated as follows.

- u_2 is normalized by k_2 in eq. (5.19). Therefore, we take $u_{20} = k_2 = 5 \times 10^{-6}$ M.

TABLE 2.6 Parameters in eqs. (2.6).

Parameter	Value
k_1	3.9×10^{-9} M cm^2 sec^{-1}
k_2	5×10^{-6} M
k_3	1.62×10^{-9} hr ml^{-1} cell^{-1}
k_4	3.5×10^{8} cells ml^{-1}
k_9	4×10^{-6} M^2
D_1	$2 - 4 \times 10^{-6}$ cm^2 s^{-1}
D_2	8.9×10^{-6} cm^2 s^{-1}
D_3	$\approx 9 \times 10^{-6}$ cm^2 s^{-1}
u_{10}	10^9 cells ml^{-1}
u_{30}	$1 - 3 \times 10^{-3}$ M

- From the term $\frac{u_1^2}{k_6 + u_1^2}$ in eq. (2.6b), for $k_6 \approx u_1^2$, we take $k_6 = u_{10}^2 = 10^{18}$.
- From the term $\frac{u_3^2}{k_9 + u_3^2}$ in eq. (2.6c), for $k_9 \approx u_3^2$, we take $k_9 = u_{30}^2 = 10^{-6}$ (adjusted to $k_9 = 4 \times 10^{-6}$).
- From the term $k_5 u_3 \frac{u_1^2}{k_6 + u_1^2}$ in eq. (2.6b), if $\frac{\partial u_2}{\partial t} \approx 5 \times 10^{-9}$ M s^{-1}, we take $k_5(1 \times 10^{-3}) = 5 \times 10^{-9}$ or $k_5 = 5 \times 10^{-6}$ (adjusted to $k_5 = 5 \times 10^{-7}$).
- From the term $k_7 u_1 u_2$ in eq. (2.6b), we take $(k_7)(10^9)(5 \times 10^{-6}) = 5 \times 10^{-9}$ or $k_7 = 10^{-12}$ (adjusted to $k_7 = 10^{-13}$).
- From the term $k_8 u_1 \frac{u_3^2}{k_9 + u_3^2}$ in eq. (2.6c), if $\frac{\partial u_3}{\partial t} \approx 10^{-6}$ M s^{-1}, we take $k_8(10^9) = 10^{-6}$ or $k_8 = 10^{-15}$ (adjusted to $k_8 = 10^{-14}$).

In this way, u_{20}, k_5, k_6, k_7, and k_8 are estimated by an order-of-magnitude analysis and assumed values of the LHS derivatives of eqs. (2.6b) and (2.6c), followed possibly by some adjustment (and are not estimated from physical/chemical considerations or data). As a detail, the designation M in Table 2.6 is taken as molar, that is, M = gmol/cm^3 = gmol/ml where g is gram.

Eqs. (2.6) each require an IC and two BCs. The IC for all three PDEs is taken as a Gaussian function.

$$u_1(x,t=0) = u_{10}e^{-\lambda x^2}; \; u_2(x,t=0) = u_{20}e^{-\lambda x^2};$$
$$u_3(x,t=0) = u_{30}e^{-\lambda x^2} \tag{2.7a,b,c}$$

where u_{10}, u_{20}, u_{30}, and λ are constants to be specified.

The zero-flux BCs (2.4) are again used for the three PDEs.

$$\frac{\partial u_1(x=0,t)}{\partial x} = \frac{\partial u_1(x=L,t)}{\partial x} = 0 \tag{2.8a,b}$$

$$\frac{\partial u_2(x=0,t)}{\partial x} = \frac{\partial u_2(x=L,t)}{\partial x} = 0 \tag{2.8c,d}$$

$$\frac{\partial u_3(x=0,t)}{\partial x} = \frac{\partial u_3(x=L,t)}{\partial x} = 0 \tag{2.8e,f}$$

Eqs. (2.6) to (2.8) constitute the 3-PDE model. We now consider the numerical solution of these equations, starting with the ODE routine based on the method of lines (MOL).

2.3.1 ODE Routine

The following ODE routine for eqs. (2.6) and (2.8) parallels the 2-PDE ODE routine of Listing 2.1 (Listing 2.3 next).

```
  p_form_2=function(t,u,parms){
#
# Function p_form_2 computes the t derivative vector of
# the u1, u2, u3 vectors
#
# One vector to three vectors
  u1=rep(0,nx);u2=rep(0,nx);u3=rep(0,nx);
  for(i in 1:nx){
    u1[i]=u[i];
    u2[i]=u[i+nx];
    u3[i]=u[i+2*nx];
  }
#
# u1x, u2x, u3x
  u1x=dss004(xl,xu,nx,u1);
  u2x=dss004(xl,xu,nx,u2);
  u3x=dss004(xl,xu,nx,u3);
#
# Boundary conditions
  u1x[1]=0;u1x[nx]=0;
  u2x[1]=0;u2x[nx]=0;
  u3x[1]=0;u3x[nx]=0;
  nl=2;nu=2;
#
# u1xx, u2xx, u3xx
  u1xx=dss044(xl,xu,nx,u1,u1x,nl,nu);
  u2xx=dss044(xl,xu,nx,u2,u2x,nl,nu);
  u3xx=dss044(xl,xu,nx,u3,u3x,nl,nu);
#
# RHS terms
  term1=rep(0,nx);term2=rep(0,nx);term3=rep(0,nx);
  for(i in 1:nx){
```

```
    den=1/(k[2]+u2[i])^2;
    term1[i]=k[1]*u1[i]*den*u2xx[i];
    term2[i]=k[1]*den*u1x[i]*u2x[i];
    term3[i]=-2*k[1]*u1[i]*den/(k[2]+u2[i])*u2x[i]^2;
  {
#
# PDEs
  u1t=rep(0,nx);u2t=rep(0,nx);u3t=rep(0,nx);
  for(i in 1:nx){
    u1t[i]=D1*u1xx[i]-(term1[i]+term2[i]+term3[i])+
           k[3]*u1[i]*(k[4]*u3[i]^2/(k[9]+u3[i]^2)-u1[i]);
    u2t[i]=D2*u2xx[i]+k[5]*u3[i]*(u1[i]^2/(k[6]+u1[i]^2)-
           k[7]*u1[i]*u2[i]);
    u3t[i]=D3*u3xx[i]-k[8]*u1[i]*(u3[i]^2/(k[9]+u3[i]^2));
  }
#
# Three vectors to one vector
  ut=rep(0,3*nx);
  for(i in 1:nx){
    ut[i]     =u1t[i];
    ut[i+nx]  =u2t[i];
    ut[i+2*nx]=u3t[i];
  }
#
# Increment calls to p_form_2
  ncall <<- ncall+1;
#
# Return derivative vector
  return(list(c(ut)));
}
```

Listing 2.3 ODE routine p_form_2.

We can note the following details about p_form_2.

- The function is defined.

```
    p_form_2=function(t,u,parms){
  #
  # Function p_form_2 computes the t derivative vector
  # of the u1, u2, u3 vectors
```

The input arguments are in conformity with the R ODE integrators, in this case `lsodes` called by the main program discussed subsequently. `lsodes` in turn calls `p_form_2`. For the number of points in x, `nx=51`, `u` is a vector of `(3)(nx)=(3)(51)=153` elements, that is, `51` points in x for each of eqs. (2.6) (`153` ODEs in the MOL approximation of eqs. (2.6)). `nx` is defined numerically in the main program discussed subsequently. `parms` is unused.

- `u` is placed in three vectors, `u1,u2,u3`, to facilitate subsequent programming in terms of problem oriented variables, that is, the dependent variables of eqs. (2.6).

```
#
# One vector to three vectors
  u1=rep(0,nx);u2=rep(0,nx);u3=rep(0,nx);
  for(i in 1:nx){
    u1[i]=u[i];
    u2[i]=u[i+nx];
    u3[i]=u[i+2*nx];
  }
```

Note the ease with which a PDE can be added to the 2-PDE model of eqs. (2.2).

- $\partial u_1/\partial x, \partial u_2/\partial x, \partial u_3/\partial x$ are computed by the library differentiator `dss004`. `xl,xu` are set in the main program.

```
#
# u1x, u2x, u3x
  u1x=dss004(xl,xu,nx,u1);
  u2x=dss004(xl,xu,nx,u2);
  u3x=dss004(xl,xu,nx,u3);
```

- BCs (2.8) are programmed.

```
#
# Boundary conditions
  u1x[1]=0;u1x[nx]=0;
  u2x[1]=0;u2x[nx]=0;
  u3x[1]=0;u3x[nx]=0;
  nl=2;nu=2;
```

Again, since the BCs specify the partial derivatives at the boundaries, that is, $\partial u_1(x=0,t)/\partial x = 0$, $\partial u_1(x=L,t)/\partial x = 0$, and similar conditions for u_2, u_3, Neumann BCs are designated with `nl,nu`.

- $\partial^2 u_1/\partial x^2, \partial^2 u_2/\partial x^2, \partial^2 u_3/\partial x^2$ are computed by the library differentiator `dss044`.

```
#
# u1xx, u2xx, u3xx
  u1xx=dss044(xl,xu,nx,u1,u1x,nl,nu);
  u2xx=dss044(xl,xu,nx,u2,u2x,nl,nu);
  u3xx=dss044(xl,xu,nx,u3,u3x,nl,nu);
```

Note that the derivatives at the boundaries, `u1x[1],u1x[nx]`, `u2x[1],u2x[nx]`, and `u3x[1],u3x[nx]`, are inputs to `dss044`.

- The programming of three RHS terms of eq. (2.6a) is similar to the previous programming of eq. (2.5). A `for` with index `i` is used for the interval $0 \le x \le L$.

```
#
# RHS terms
  term1=rep(0,nx);term2=rep(0,nx);term3=rep(0,nx);
  for(i in 1:nx){
    den=1/(k[2]+u2[i])^2;
    term1[i]=k[1]*u1[i]*den*u2xx[i];
    term2[i]=k[1]*den*u1x[i]*u2x[i];
    term3[i]=-2*k[1]*u1[i]*den/(k[2]+u2[i])*u2x[i]^2;
  }
```

- Eqs (2.6) are programmed in a `for` with index `i`.

```
#
# PDEs
  u1t=rep(0,nx);u2t=rep(0,nx);u3t=rep(0,nx);
  for(i in 1:nx){
    u1t[i]=D1*u1xx[i]-(term1[i]+term2[i]+term3[i])+
              k[3]*u1[i]*(k[4]*u3[i]^2/(k[9]+u3[i]^2)
                 -u1[i]);
    u2t[i]=D2*u2xx[i]+k[5]*u3[i]*(u1[i]^2/(k[6]+
       u1[i]^2)-k[7]*u1[i]*u2[i]);
```

```
    u3t[i]=D3*u3xx[i]-k[8]*u1[i]*(u3[i]^2/(k[9]+
       u3[i]^2));
  }
```

$D_1, D_2, D_3, k_3, k_4, k_5, k_6, k_7, k_8, k_9$ are defined numerically in the main program. The derivatives $\partial u_1/\partial t, \partial u_2/\partial t, \partial u_3/\partial t$ in u1t,u2t,u3t are the final result. They are passed to lsodes for the integration of the 153 ODEs.

- The derivatives u1t,u2t,u3t are placed in a single vector ut that is returned to lsodes for the integration of the 153 ODEs.

```
#
# Three vectors to one vector
  ut=rep(0,3*nx);
  for(i in 1:nx){
    ut[i]      =u1t[i];
    ut[i+nx]   =u2t[i];
    ut[i+2*nx]=u3t[i];
  }
```

An important check is that the number of dependent variable (e.g., in u) equals the number of derivatives (e.g., in ut) and that each dependent variable and its associated derivative are in the same positions in the dependent variable and derivative vectors. While this positioning is rather obvious in the present case, generally for models with relatively large numbers of ODEs, the correct positioning may not be so obvious and, of course, even one dependent variable misplaced with respect to its derivative will produce an incorrect solution.

- The number of calls to p_form_2 is incremented and the value returned to the main program with <<-. The derivative vector is then returned from p_form_2 as a list (as required by the R ODE integrators including lsodes).

```
#
# Increment calls to p_form_2
  ncall <<- ncall+1;
```

```
#
# Return derivative vector
  return(list(c(ut)));
}
```

The final } concludes p_form_2.

In summary, the model consisting of eqs. (2.6) and (2.8) is programmed in p_form_2. The only part of the model not included in this routine are the ICs for eqs. (2.6), that is, eqs. (2.7), to start the numerical solution. We now consider the effect of different parameter sets and some features of the numerical and graphical outputs produced by the main program. In addition, the RHS terms of eqs. (2.6) are computed and displayed to give further insight into the origin of various features of the PDE solutions.

2.3.2 Main Program

The main program that calls p_form_2 of Listing 2.3 through lsodes is similar to the main program of Listing 2.2.

```
#
# Access ODE integrator
  library("deSolve");
#
# Access functions for analytical solutions
  setwd("c:/R/bme_pde/chap2/v_3pde");
  source("p_form_2.R");
  source("pde_terms.R");
  source("dss004.R");
  source("dss044.R");
#
# Level of output
#
#   ip = 1 - graphical (plotted) solutions
#            (u1(x,t), u2(x,t), u3(x,t)) only
#
#   ip = 2 - numerical and graphical solutions
#
  ip=2;
```

```
#
# Parameters
#
# ncase = 1: Fickian diffusion
#
# ncase = 2: Fickian diffusion
#
#            Chemotaxis diffusion
#
# ncase = 3: Fickian diffusion
#
#            Chemotaxis diffusion
#
#            Source term in u1 PDE
#
# ncase = 4: Fickian diffusion
#
#            Chemotaxis diffusion
#
#            Source term in u1 PDE
#
#            Source term in u2 PDE
#
# ncase = 5: Fickian diffusion
#
#            Chemotaxis diffusion
#
#            Source term in u1 PDE
#
#            Source term in u2 PDE
#
#            Source term in u3 PDE
#
# ncase = 6: ncase = 5 plus the LHS and RHS terms of the
#            three pdes
#
#            Seven PDE RHS terms in chemo1 to chemo7
#
#            Three PDE LHS (derivatives in t) in
#            chemo8 to chemo10
#
```

```
  ncase=6;
#
# ncase = 1
  if(ncase==1){
    D1=2.0e-06;D2=8.9e-06;D3=9.0e-06;
    k=rep(0,9);
  }
#
# ncase = 2
  if(ncase==2){
    D1=2.0e-06;D2=8.9e-06;D3=9.0e-06;
    k=rep(0,9);
    k[1]=3.9e-09;k[2]=5.0e-06;
  }
#
# ncase = 3
  if(ncase==3){
    D1=2.0e-06;D2=8.9e-06;D3=9.0e-06;
    k=rep(0,9);
    k[1]=3.9e-09;k[2]=5.0e-06;k[3]=1.62e-09;
    k[4]=3.5e+08;k[9]=4.0e-06;
  }
#
# ncase = 4
  if(ncase==4){
    D1=2.0e-06;D2=8.9e-06;D3=9.0e-06;
    k=rep(0,9);
    k[1]=3.9e-09;k[2]=5.0e-06;k[3]=1.62e-09;
    k[4]=3.5e+08;k[9]=4.0e-06;
    k[5]=5.0e-07;k[6]=1.0e+18;k[7]=1.0e-13;
  }
#
# ncase = 5, 6
  if(ncase==5 || ncase==6){
    D1=2.0e-06;D2=8.9e-06;D3=9.0e-06;
    k=rep(0,9);
    k[1]=3.9e-09;k[2]=5.0e-06;k[3]=1.62e-09;
    k[4]=3.5e+08;k[9]= 4.0e-06;
    k[5]=5.0e-07;k[6]=1.0e+18;k[7]=1.0e-13;
    k[8]=1.0e-14;
  }
```

```
#
# Write parameters
  cat(sprintf("\n\n D1 = %8.3e  D2 = %8.3e  D3 = %8.3e \n",
          D1,D2,D3));
#
# Write heading
  if(ip==1){
    cat(sprintf("\n Graphical output only\n"));
  }
#
# Grid (in x)
  nx=51;xl=0;xu=1;
  xg=seq(from=xl,to=xu,by=0.02);
#
# Independent variable for ODE integration
  nout=11;
  tout=seq(from=0,to=5*3600,by=0.5*3600);
#
# Initial condition
  u0=rep(0,3*nx);
  u10=1.0e+08;u20=5.0e-06;u30=1.0e-03;
  for(i in 1:nx){
    u0[i]     =u10*exp(-5*xg[i]^2);
    u0[i+nx]  =u20*exp(-5*xg[i]^2);
    u0[i+2*nx]=u30*exp(-5*xg[i]^2);
  }
  t=0;
  ncall=0;
#
# ODE integration
  out=lsodes(y=u0,times=tout,func=p_form_2,parms=NULL)
  nrow(out)
  ncol(out)
#
# Arrays for plotting numerical solution
  u1_plot=matrix(0,nrow=nx,ncol=nout);
  u2_plot=matrix(0,nrow=nx,ncol=nout);
  u3_plot=matrix(0,nrow=nx,ncol=nout);
  for(it in 1:nout){
    for(ix in 1:nx){
       u1_plot[ix,it]=out[it,ix+1];
```

```
      u2_plot[ix,it]=out[it,ix+1+nx];
      u3_plot[ix,it]=out[it,ix+1+2*nx];
    }
  }
#
# Display numerical solution
  if(ip==2){
    for(it in 1:nout){
      cat(sprintf(
      "\n      t       x     u1(x,t)     u2(x,t)
         u3(x,t)\n"));
      for(ix in 1:nx){
        cat(sprintf("%7.2f%8.3f%12.3e%12.3e%12.3e\n",
        tout[it]/3600,xg[ix],u1_plot[ix,it],u2_plot[ix,it],
                           u3_plot[ix,it]));
      }
    }
  }
#
# Calls to ODE routine
  cat(sprintf("\n\n ncall = %5d\n\n",ncall));
#
# Plot u1
  par(mfrow=c(1,1));
  matplot(x=xg,y=u1_plot,type="l",xlab="x",
          ylab="u1(x,t), t=0,0.5,...,5",xlim=c(xl,xu),
             lty=1,main="u1(x,t); t=0,0.5,...,5;",lwd=2);
#
# Plot u2
  par(mfrow=c(1,1));
  matplot(x=xg,y=u2_plot,type="l",xlab="x",
          ylab="u2(x,t), t=0,0.5,...,5",xlim=c(xl,xu),
             lty=1,main="u2(x,t); t=0,0.5,...,5;",lwd=2);
#
# Plot u3
  par(mfrow=c(1,1));
  matplot(x=xg,y=u3_plot,type="l",xlab="x",
          ylab="u3(x,t), t=0,0.5,...,5",xlim=c(xl,xu),
             lty=1,main="u3(x,t); t=0,0.5,...,5;",lwd=2);
#
# Supplemental calculations
```

```
  if(ncase==6){
    chemo1_2d=matrix(0,nrow=nx,ncol=nout);
    chemo2_2d=matrix(0,nrow=nx,ncol=nout);
    chemo3_2d=matrix(0,nrow=nx,ncol=nout);
    chemo4_2d=matrix(0,nrow=nx,ncol=nout);
    chemo5_2d=matrix(0,nrow=nx,ncol=nout);
    chemo6_2d=matrix(0,nrow=nx,ncol=nout);
    chemo7_2d=matrix(0,nrow=nx,ncol=nout);
    chemo8_2d=matrix(0,nrow=nx,ncol=nout);
    chemo9_2d=matrix(0,nrow=nx,ncol=nout);
   chemo10_2d=matrix(0,nrow=nx,ncol=nout);
#
#   Step through t
    for(it in 1:nout){
      pde_terms(tout[it],c(u1_plot[,it],u2_plot[,it],
                           u3_plot[,it]));
      chemo1_2d[,it]=chemo1; chemo2_2d[,it]=chemo2;
      chemo3_2d[,it]=chemo3; chemo4_2d[,it]=chemo4;
      chemo5_2d[,it]=chemo5; chemo6_2d[,it]=chemo6;
      chemo7_2d[,it]=chemo7; chemo8_2d[,it]=chemo8;
      chemo9_2d[,it]=chemo9;chemo10_2d[,it]=chemo10;
    }
#
# Plot chemo1 (D1*u1_xx)
  par(mfrow=c(1,1));
  matplot(x=xg,y=chemo1_2d[,-1],type="l",xlab="x",
          ylab="D1*u1_{xx}, t=0.5,...,5",xlim=c(xl,xu),
             lty=1,main="D1*u1_{xx}; t=0.5,...,5;",lwd=2);
#
# Plot chemo8 (u1_t)
  par(mfrow=c(1,1));
  matplot(x=xg,y=chemo8_2d[,-1],type="l",xlab="x",
          ylab="u1_t, t=0.5,...,5",xlim=c(xl,xu),lty=1,
          main="u1_t; t=0.5,...,5;",lwd=2);
#
# Plot chemo9 (u2_t)
  par(mfrow=c(1,1));
  matplot(x=xg,y=chemo9_2d[,-1],type="l",xlab="x",
          ylab="u2_t, t=0.5,...,5",xlim=c(xl,xu),lty=1,
```

```
          main="u2_t; t=0.5,...,5;",lwd=2);
#
# Plot chemo10 (u3_t)
  par(mfrow=c(1,1));
  matplot(x=xg,y=chemo10_2d[,-1],type="l",xlab="x",
          ylab="u3_t, t=0.5,...,5",xlim=c(xl,xu),lty=1,
          main="u3_t; t=0.5,...,5;",lwd=2);
```

Listing 2.4 Main program for eqs. (2.6).

We can note the following points about this main program (with emphasis on the details pertaining to eqs. (2.6)).

- `p_form_2` of Listing 2.3 is accessed.

```
  setwd("c:/R/bme_pde/chap2/v_3pde");
  source("p_form_2.R");
```

- The level of output is specified with `ip` as in Listing 2.2. Then, six cases pertaining to parameter changes are programmed. For the subsequent discussion, `ncase=6` is used.

```
#
# ncase = 5, 6
  if(ncase==5 || ncase==6){
    D1=2.0e-06;D2=8.9e-06;D3=9.0e-06;
    k=rep(0,9);
    k[1]=3.9e-09;k[2]=5.0e-06;k[3]=1.62e-09;
    k[4]=3.5e+08;k[9]= 4.0e-06;
    k[5]=5.0e-07;k[6]=1.0e+18;k[7]=1.0e-13;
    k[8]=1.0e-14;
  }
```

The `or` operator in R is `||`. The nine elements of the rate constant vector `k` are given specific values (in contrast with `ncase=1,2,3,4` for which some of the zero default values are used). Also, for `ncase=6`, the RHS terms of eqs. (2.6) are computed and displayed (discussed subsequently).

- The grid in x is defined as $0 \leq x \leq 1$, with 51 points so that $x = 0, 0.02, \ldots, 1$.

```
#
# Grid (in x)
  nx=51;xl=0;xu=1;
  xg=seq(from=xl,to=xu,by=0.02);
```

- The interval in t is $0 \leq t \leq (5)(3600)$ s (seconds), corresponding to a total interval of 5 h, with 11 values, $t = 0, (0.5)(3600), \ldots, (5)(3600)$, for the output.

```
#
# Independent variable for ODE integration
  nout=11;
  tout=seq(from=0,to=5*3600,by=0.5*3600);
```

  The basic unit of time t for the calculations is s (seconds) because the model parameters are in s as listed in Table 2.6.

- Three ICs for eqs. (2.6) are Gaussian functions in accordance with eqs. (2.7).

```
#
# Initial condition
  u0=rep(0,3*nx);
  u10=1.0e+08;u20=5.0e-06;u30=1.0e-03;
  for(i in 1:nx){
    u0[i]     =u10*exp(-5*xg[i]^2);
    u0[i+nx]  =u20*exp(-5*xg[i]^2);
    u0[i+2*nx]=u30*exp(-5*xg[i]^2);
  }
  t=0;
  ncall=0;
```

  Note that u10=1.0e+08 and u20=5.0e-06 so that the dependent variables range over approximately 14 orders of magnitude. But even with this wide variation in magnitude, lsodes is able to compute a numerical solution to eqs. (2.6). Also, this large range illustrates a common difference between dimensional variables such as u_1, u_2, u_3 of eqs. (2.6) and dimensionless variables such as u_1, u_2 of eqs. (2.2); the latter are often normalized to have values close to 1.

- The ODEs are integrated by lsodes, which is informed of the number of ODEs ((3)(51)=153) by the length of the IC vector u0. Also, the output vector tout has length 11 (programmed previously).

```
#
# ODE integration
  out=lsodes(y=u0,times=tout,func=p_form_2,parms=NULL)
  nrow(out)
  ncol(out
```

Note the use of the ODE routine p_form_2 of Listing 2.3.

- The solution is put into three 2D arrays, u1_plot,u2_plot, u3_plot, for subsequent plotting.

```
#
# Arrays for plotting numerical solution
  u1_plot=matrix(0,nrow=nx,ncol=nout);
  u2_plot=matrix(0,nrow=nx,ncol=nout);
  u3_plot=matrix(0,nrow=nx,ncol=nout);
  for(it in 1:nout){
    for(ix in 1:nx){
       u1_plot[ix,it]=out[it,ix+1];
       u2_plot[ix,it]=out[it,ix+1+nx];
       u3_plot[ix,it]=out[it,ix+1+2*nx];
    }
  }
```

Note again the offset of 1 in the second subscript of out, for example, ix+1, because the values of t are included in out as out[it,1]. Thus, out has the dimensions out[nout,3*nx+1]= out[11,3*51+1]=out[11,154].

- For ip=2, the numerical solution is displayed in tabular form.

```
#
# Display numerical solution
  if(ip==2){
    for(it in 1:nout){
      cat(sprintf(
      "\n   t      x   u1(x,t)   u2(x,t)   u3(x,t)\n"));
```

```
      for(ix in 1:nx){
        cat(sprintf("%7.2f%8.3f%12.3e%12.3e%12.3e\n",
        tout[it]/3600,xg[ix],u1_plot[ix,it],u2_plot
           [ix,it],u3_plot[ix,it]));
      }
    }
  }
```

t in `tout` is converted to hours before it is displayed. Also, the `%12.3e` format is used because of the wide variation in the magnitude of the three dependent variables u_1, u_2, u_3 as discussed previously.

- The number of calls to `p_form_2` is displayed at the end of the solution as a measure of the computational effort to compute the solution. Then, u_1, u_2, u_3 are plotted separately by using `par(mfrow=c(1,1))`.

```
#
# Plot u1
  par(mfrow=c(1,1));
  matplot(x=xg,y=u1_plot,type="l",xlab="x",
          ylab="u1(x,t), t=0,0.5,...,5",xlim=c(xl,xu),
             lty=1,main="u1(x,t); t=0,0.5,...,5;",
                lwd=2);

    etc. for u2, u3
```

- For `ncase=6`, `10` arrays are declared (preallocated) for various terms in eqs. (2.6). Two-dimensional arrays are used to facilitate subsequent plotting.

```
#
# Supplemental calculations
  if(ncase==6){
    chemo1_2d=matrix(0,nrow=nx,ncol=nout);
    chemo2_2d=matrix(0,nrow=nx,ncol=nout);
    chemo3_2d=matrix(0,nrow=nx,ncol=nout);
    chemo4_2d=matrix(0,nrow=nx,ncol=nout);
    chemo5_2d=matrix(0,nrow=nx,ncol=nout);
    chemo6_2d=matrix(0,nrow=nx,ncol=nout);
```

```
   chemo7_2d=matrix(0,nrow=nx,ncol=nout);
   chemo8_2d=matrix(0,nrow=nx,ncol=nout);
   chemo9_2d=matrix(0,nrow=nx,ncol=nout);
  chemo10_2d=matrix(0,nrow=nx,ncol=nout);
```

As an incidental programming note, two or more of these matrix statements could be placed in individual lines, but then the lines would be too long for listing and printing.

- A call to routine pde_terms (discussed subsequently) computes the values of the 10 terms chemo1 to chemo10 (returned from pde_terms). The for with index it is used for the nout=11 values of t in the interval $0 \leq t \leq (5)(3600)$.

```
#
#   Step through t
    for(it in 1:nout){
      pde_terms(tout[it],c(u1_plot[,it],u2_plot[,it],
                           u3_plot[,it]));
      chemo1_2d[,it]=chemo1; chemo2_2d[,it]=chemo2;
      chemo3_2d[,it]=chemo3; chemo4_2d[,it]=chemo4;
      chemo5_2d[,it]=chemo5; chemo6_2d[,it]=chemo6;
      chemo7_2d[,it]=chemo7; chemo8_2d[,it]=chemo8;
      chemo9_2d[,it]=chemo9;chemo10_2d[,it]=chemo10;
    }
```

The 10 terms are then placed in the 2D arrays. pde_terms performs the derivative calculations of p_form_2, but it also computes the 10 terms so that it is provided as a separate routine (i.e., a call to p_form_1 alone would not be sufficient). Also, note the use of the [,it] subscripts for the 51 values of x at each value of t.

- The 10 terms could all be plotted, but here only four are selected, chemo1, chem08, chemo9, and chemo10.

```
#
# Plot chemo1 (D1*u1_xx)
  par(mfrow=c(1,1));
  matplot(x=xg,y=chemo1_2d[,-1],type="l",xlab="x",
          ylab="D1*u1_{xx}, t=0.5,...,5",xlim=c(xl,xu),
```

```
                lty=1,main="D1*u1_{xx}; t=0.5,...,5;",
                   lwd=2);

      etc. for chemo8, chemo9, chemo10
```

This level of output illustrates how PDEs can be studied in detail (rather than just considering the dependent variables, such as $u_1(x,t), u_2(x,t), u_3(x,t)$, as a function of the independent variables, such as x, t).

Note also that the first subscript in t is not used in the plotting of chem01,chemo8,chemo9,chemo10, that is, t starts at $t = 0.5$ rather than $t = 0$. For example, chemo1_2d[,-1] excludes [,1]. The reason for this form of plotting to exclude $t = 0$ is to avoid the discontinuity between the ICs of eqs. (2.7) and the BCs of eqs. (2.8) (at $x = 0, x = L = 1$). For $t > 0$, this discontinuity is smoothed (by diffusion) and therefore does not produce a disruption in the plotting (the reader could try chemo1_2d to observe the output at $t = 0$).

The routine pde_terms for the calculation of the 10 terms chemo1 to chemo10 follows next.

2.3.3 Supplemental Routine

pde_terms in Listing 2.5 calculates the 10 RHS terms chemo1 to chem10 for the plotting in the main program of Listing 2.4 discussed previously.

```
  pde_terms=function(t,u){
#
# Function pde_terms provides supplemental calculations
#    for the three-pde
# model based on the u1, u2, u3 vectors
#
# One vector to three vectors
  u1=rep(0,nx);u2=rep(0,nx);u3=rep(0,nx);
  for(i in 1:nx){
    u1[i]=u[i];
    u2[i]=u[i+nx];
```

```
    u3[i]=u[i+2*nx];
  }
#
# u1x, u2x
  u1x=dss004(xl,xu,nx,u1);
  u2x=dss004(xl,xu,nx,u2);
  u3x=dss004(xl,xu,nx,u3);
#
# Boundary conditions
  u1x[1]=0;u1x[nx]=0;
  u2x[1]=0;u2x[nx]=0;
  u3x[1]=0;u3x[nx]=0;
  nl=2;nu=2;
#
# u1xx, u2xx
  u1xx=dss044(xl,xu,nx,u1,u1x,nl,nu);
  u2xx=dss044(xl,xu,nx,u2,u2x,nl,nu);
  u3xx=dss044(xl,xu,nx,u3,u3x,nl,nu);
#
# RHS terms
  term1=rep(0,nx);term2=rep(0,nx);term3=rep(0,nx);
  for(i in 1:nx){
    den=1/(k[2]+u2[i])^2;
    term1[i]=k[1]*u1[i]*den*u2xx[i];
    term2[i]=k[1]*den*u1x[i]*u2x[i];
    term3[i]=-2*k[1]*u1[i]*den/(k[2]+u2[i])*u2x[i]^2;
  }
#
# PDEs
  u1t=rep(0,nx);u2t=rep(0,nx);u3t=rep(0,nx);
  for(i in 1:nx){
    u1t[i]=D1*u1xx[i]-(term1[i]+term2[i]+term3[i])+
           k[3]*u1[i]*(k[4]*u3[i]^2/(k[9]+u3[i]^2)-u1[i]);
    u2t[i]=D2*u2xx[i]+k[5]*u3[i]*(u1[i]^2/(k[6]+u1[i]^2)-
           k[7]*u1[i]*u2[i]);
    u3t[i]=D3*u3xx[i]-k[8]*u1[i]*(u3[i]^2/(k[9]+u3[i]^2));
  }
#
# PDE terms
  chemo1=rep(0,nx);chemo2=rep(0,nx);chemo3=rep(0,nx);
  chemo4=rep(0,nx);chemo5=rep(0,nx);chemo6=rep(0,nx);
```

```
  chemo7=rep(0,nx);chemo8=rep(0,nx);chemo9=rep(0,nx);
 chemo10=rep(0,nx);
  for(i in 1:nx){
    chemo1[i]=D1*u1xx[i];
    chemo2[i]=-(term1[i]+term2[i]+term3[i]);
    chemo3[i]=k[3]*u1[i]*(k[4]*u3[i]^2/(k[9]+u3[i]^2)-
       u1[i]);
    chemo4[i]=D2*u2xx[i];
    chemo5[i]=k[5]*u3[i]*(u1[i]^2/(k[6]+u1[i]^2)-k[7]
       *u1[i]*u2[i]);
    chemo6[i]=D3*u3xx[i];
    chemo7[i]=-k[8]*u1[i]*(u3[i]^2/(k[9]+u3[i]^2));
    chemo8[i]=u1t[i];
    chemo9[i]=u2t[i];
   chemo10[i]=u3t[i];
  }
#
# Return arrays of PDE terms
  chemo1 <<- chemo1;chemo2 <<- chemo2;chemo3 <<- chemo3;
  chemo4 <<- chemo4;chemo5 <<- chemo5;chemo6 <<- chemo6;
  chemo7 <<- chemo7;chemo8 <<- chemo8;chemo9 <<- chemo9;
  chemo10<<-chemo10;
}
```

Listing 2.5 pde_terms for the calculation of the terms in eqs. (2.6).

We can note the following details about pde_terms.

- pde_terms is essentially the same as p_form_2 of Listing 2.3 up to and including the calculation of the derivative vectors ut1,u2t,u3t. Then, the 10 RHS terms of eqs. (2.6) are calculated as a function of x using a for with index i.

```
#
# PDE terms
  chemo1=rep(0,nx);chemo2=rep(0,nx);chemo3=rep(0,nx);
  chemo4=rep(0,nx);chemo5=rep(0,nx);chemo6=rep(0,nx);
  chemo7=rep(0,nx);chemo8=rep(0,nx);chemo9=rep(0,nx);
 chemo10=rep(0,nx);
  for(i in 1:nx){
    chemo1[i]=D1*u1xx[i];
```

```
    chemo2[i]=-(term1[i]+term2[i]+term3[i]);
    chemo3[i]=k[3]*u1[i]*(k[4]*u3[i]^2/(k[9]+u3[i]^2)
       -u1[i]);
    chemo4[i]=D2*u2xx[i];
    chemo5[i]=k[5]*u3[i]*(u1[i]^2/(k[6]+u1[i]^2)-k[7]
       *u1[i]*u2[i]);
    chemo6[i]=D3*u3xx[i];
    chemo7[i]=-k[8]*u1[i]*(u3[i]^2/(k[9]+u3[i]^2));
    chemo8[i]=u1t[i];
    chemo9[i]=u2t[i];
   chemo10[i]=u3t[i];
  }
```

For example, the diffusion term in eq. (2.6a), $D_1 \partial^2 u_1/\partial x^2$, is calculated as `chemo1[i]=D1*u1xx[i]`. The derivatives in t, $\partial u_1/\partial t$, $\partial u_2/\partial t$, and $\partial u_3/\partial t$, are placed in `chemo8,chemo9,chemo10`, respectively. In this way, the dependent variables u_1, u_2, u_3 and their derivatives in t can be examined graphically.

- The `10` arrays are returned to the main program of Listing 2.4 by the operator <<-.

```
#
# Return arrays of PDE terms
  chemo1 <<- chemo1;chemo2 <<- chemo2;chemo3 <<-
     chemo3;
  chemo4 <<- chemo4;chemo5 <<- chemo5;chemo6 <<-
     chemo6;
  chemo7 <<- chemo7;chemo8 <<- chemo8;chemo9 <<-
     chemo9;
  chemo10<<-chemo10;
}
```

The final } concludes `pde_terms`. Note that the derivative vector of `p_form_2` in Listing 2.3, `ut`, is not formed and returned as a list (`pde_terms` is not used for the numerical integration of the `153` ODEs).

This concludes the programming of eqs. (2.6) to (2.8). The numerical and graphical outputs are reviewed next.

TABLE 2.7 Abbreviated output from Listing 2.4 with ncase=6.

```
D1 = 2.000e-06  D2 = 8.900e-06  D3 = 9.000e-06

> nrow(out)
[1] 11
> ncol(out)
[1] 154

     t        x      u1(x,t)      u2(x,t)      u3(x,t)
  0.00    0.000    1.000e+08    5.000e-06    1.000e-03
  0.00    0.020    9.980e+07    4.990e-06    9.980e-04
  0.00    0.040    9.920e+07    4.960e-06    9.920e-04
  0.00    0.060    9.822e+07    4.911e-06    9.822e-04
  0.00    0.080    9.685e+07    4.843e-06    9.685e-04
  0.00    0.100    9.512e+07    4.756e-06    9.512e-04
              .                      .
              .                      .
              .                      .
     Output from x = 0.120 to 0.880 removed
              .                      .
              .                      .
              .                      .
  0.00    0.900    1.742e+06    8.711e-08    1.742e-05
  0.00    0.920    1.452e+06    7.262e-08    1.452e-05
  0.00    0.940    1.206e+06    6.029e-08    1.206e-05
  0.00    0.960    9.972e+05    4.986e-08    9.972e-06
  0.00    0.980    8.213e+05    4.107e-08    8.213e-06
  0.00    1.000    6.738e+05    3.369e-08    6.738e-06
              .                      .
              .                      .
              .                      .
     Output from t = 0.5 to 4.5 removed
              .                      .
              .                      .
              .                      .
     t        x      u1(x,t)      u2(x,t)      u3(x,t)
  5.00    0.000    1.034e+07    2.480e-06    3.449e-04
  5.00    0.020    1.034e+07    2.479e-06    3.448e-04
  5.00    0.040    1.032e+07    2.476e-06    3.445e-04
  5.00    0.060    1.029e+07    2.471e-06    3.440e-04
```

TABLE 2.7 (*Continued*)

```
  5.00   0.080   1.025e+07   2.464e-06   3.434e-04
  5.00   0.100   1.020e+07   2.455e-06   3.426e-04
                 .                       .
                 .                       .
                 .                       .
      Output from x = 0.120 to 0.880 removed
                 .                       .
                 .                       .
                 .                       .
  5.00   0.900   4.944e+06   1.505e-06   2.465e-04
  5.00   0.920   4.901e+06   1.497e-06   2.455e-04
  5.00   0.940   4.868e+06   1.490e-06   2.448e-04
  5.00   0.960   4.844e+06   1.485e-06   2.442e-04
  5.00   0.980   4.830e+06   1.482e-06   2.439e-04
  5.00   1.000   4.825e+06   1.481e-06   2.438e-04

  ncall =   831
```

2.3.4 Numerical Solution

The numerical solutions from Listings 2.3, 2.4, and 2.5 are in Table 2.7 and Figs. 2.7 to 2.13.

Table 2.7 indicates the expected variation in $t, 0 \le t \le 5$ (in hr) and $x, 0 \le x \le 1$ (in cm). Also, the large range in the dependent variables, approximately 14 orders of magnitude, is clear. The computational effort even with this large range is quite modest, `ncall = 831`.

Generally, Figs. 2.7 to 2.9 indicate that $u_1(x,t), u_2(x,t), u_3(x,t)$ have the largest variation in x at $t = 0$ and then move toward uniform values in x with increasing t. The diffusion term in eq. (2.6a), $D_1 \partial^2 u_1(x,t)/\partial x^2$, in Fig. 2.10 (`chemo01`), has a complex form but approaches a uniform zero value with increasing t. Note that $t = 0.5, \ldots, 5$ as explained previously ($t = 0$ is not included). Generally, the derivatives in t (Figs. 2.11–2.13) have the largest nonzero values at $t = 0.5$ (from the Gaussian ICs of eqs. (2.7)) and approach a uniform zero value for $u_1(x,t \to \infty), u_2(x,t \to \infty)$, $u_3(x,t \to \infty)$.

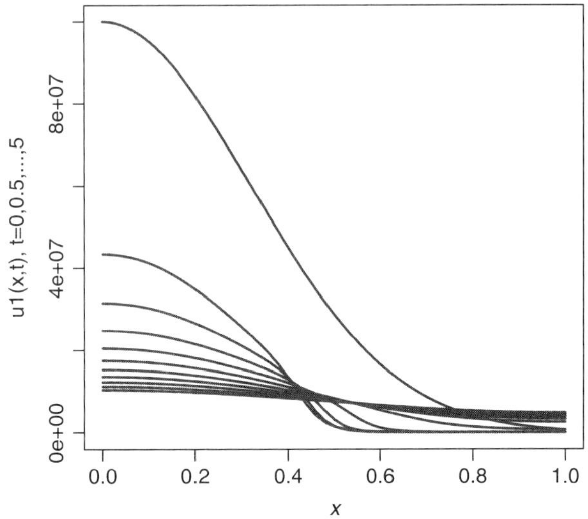

Figure 2.7 $u_1(x,t)$ versus x with t as a parameter, Gaussian IC.

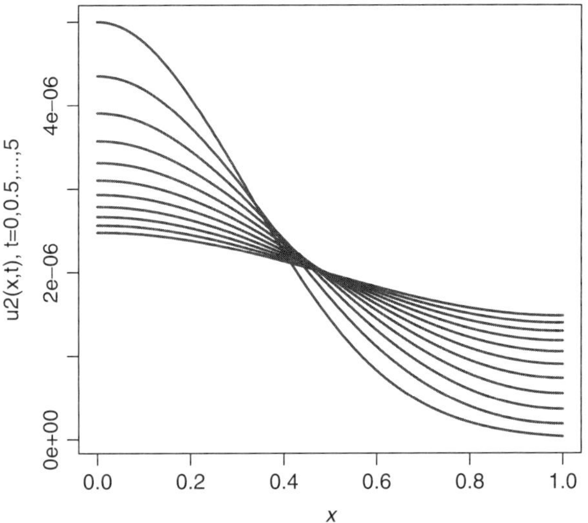

Figure 2.8 $u_2(x,t)$ versus x with t as a parameter, Gaussian IC.

In conclusion, this analysis demonstrates how PDEs can be studied in detail to understand the origin and properties of the solutions. We considered only the diffusion term in the eq. (2.6a), $D_1 \partial^2 u_1(x,t)/\partial x^2$ in Fig. 2.10, but all of the other terms in the PDEs could have

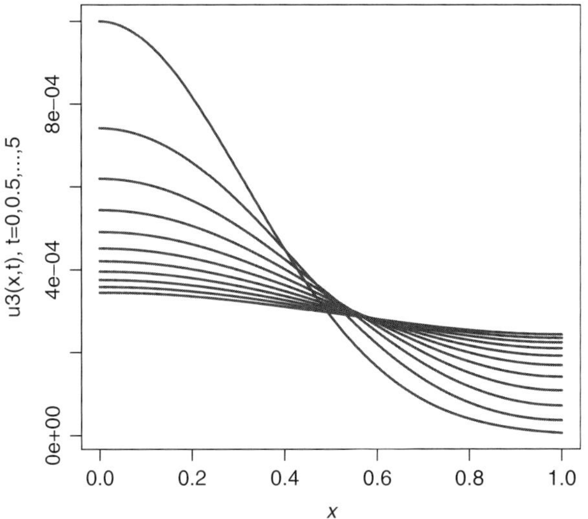

Figure 2.9 $u_3(x,t)$ versus x with t as a parameter, Gaussian IC.

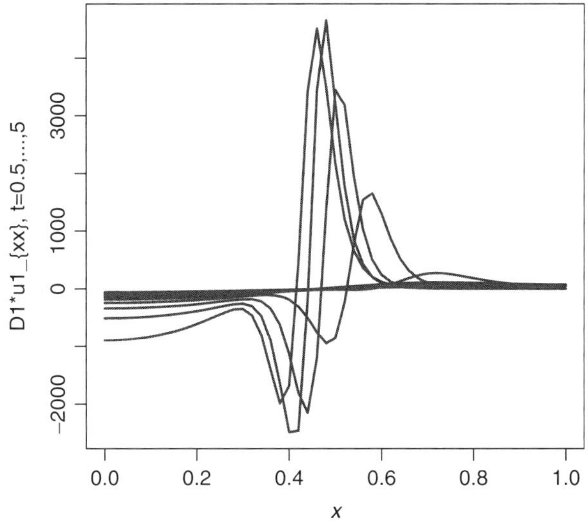

Figure 2.10 $D_1\partial^2 u_1(x,t)/\partial x^2$ versus x with $t = 0.5, \ldots, 5$ as a parameter.

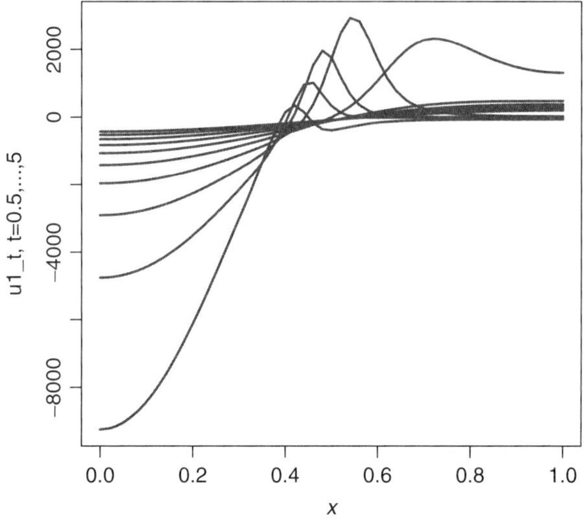

Figure 2.11 $\partial u_1(x,t)/\partial t$ versus x with $t = 0.5, \ldots, 5$ as a parameter.

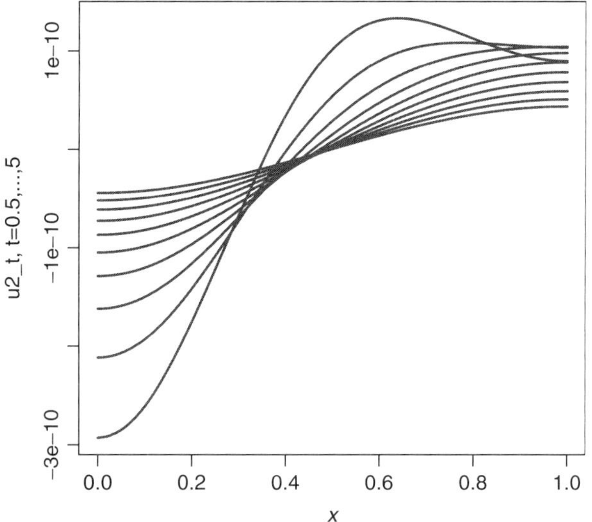

Figure 2.12 $\partial u_2(x,t)/\partial t$ versus x with $t = 0.5, \ldots, 5$ as a parameter.

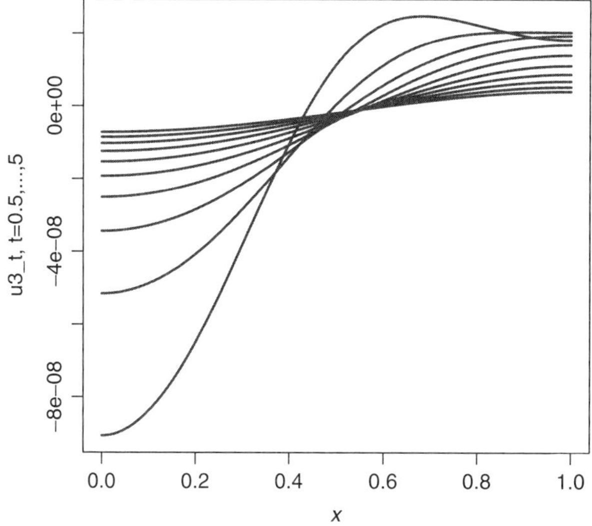

Figure 2.13 $\partial u_3(x,t)/\partial t$ versus x with $t = 0.5, \ldots, 5$ as a parameter.

been studied as well, that is, in `chemo2` to `chemo10`. Having detailed insight into the solutions generally provides guidance for the model development, revision, and interpretation, particularly for the reconciliation of the solutions with experimental data.

2.3.4.1 h Refinement The question of the accuracy of the preceding numerical solutions should also be addressed (to provide some assurance that the solutions have reasonable accuracy). To this end, we consider two procedures that can be applied without knowledge of an analytical solution (which is usually the situation for PDE models that are complicated so that analytical solutions are precluded).

First, we consider the effect of varying the number of points in x in the MOL approximation of the PDEs. This is easily achieved by changing the value of `nx` in Listing 2.4, which is accomplished, for example, with the following code.

```
#
# Grid (in x)
  nx=51;xl=0;xu=1;
  xg=seq(from=xl,to=xu,by=0.020);
```

Everything else in Listing 2.4 remains the same. We will not reconsider the previous numerical and graphical outputs for nx=51 because the solution changes very little. This is clear from the following abbreviated numerical output for the two cases, nx=41,51 (in Table 2.8).

In Table 2.8 only the solution for $x = 0, 0.1, \ldots, 1$ at $t = 5$ has been retained. The two solutions are essentially identical, suggesting nx=51 was large enough to give good accuracy. Of course, the results of Table 2.8 do not prove the level of accuracy but only imply that it is acceptable.

Also, the computational effort is reduced slightly, from ncall = 831 (nx = 51) to ncall = 754 (nx = 41). However, the reduced computation is actually more than indicated by the values of ncall because within the ODE routine p_form_2 of Listing 2.3 the number of ODEs programmed in the calculations was also reduced. This suggests that some experimentation with the parameters of a numerical algorithm, for example, nx, can be worthwhile in reducing the computational requirements while maintaining acceptable accuracy.

The preceding analysis is usually termed h *refinement* because in the numerical analysis literature, the discrete step is often denoted with h.

2.3.4.2 *p* Refinement As a second check on the accuracy, we can consider changing the order of the FD approximations of the derivatives in x in p_form_2. This is easily accomplished. For example, the fourth-order FD approximations in dss004,dss044 can be replaced with sixth-order FD approximations by using dss006,dss046. This is demonstrated with the following changes.

```
#
# u1x, u2x, u3x
  u1x=dss004(xl,xu,nx,u1);
  u2x=dss004(xl,xu,nx,u2);
  u3x=dss004(xl,xu,nx,u3);
                .
                .
                .
#
```

TABLE 2.8 Abbreviated output from Listing 2.4 with `nx=41,51`.

```
nx=41

   t        x       u1(x,t)      u2(x,t)      u3(x,t)
5.00    0.000    1.034e+07    2.480e-06    3.449e-04
5.00    0.100    1.020e+07    2.455e-06    3.426e-04
5.00    0.200    9.782e+06    2.384e-06    3.358e-04
5.00    0.300    9.137e+06    2.273e-06    3.252e-04
5.00    0.400    8.333e+06    2.133e-06    3.116e-04
5.00    0.500    7.456e+06    1.979e-06    2.961e-04
5.00    0.600    6.603e+06    1.824e-06    2.803e-04
5.00    0.700    5.860e+06    1.686e-06    2.658e-04
5.00    0.800    5.294e+06    1.576e-06    2.541e-04
5.00    0.900    4.943e+06    1.505e-06    2.465e-04
5.00    1.000    4.825e+06    1.481e-06    2.438e-04

ncall =   754

nx=51

   t        x       u1(x,t)      u2(x,t)      u3(x,t)
5.00    0.000    1.034e+07    2.480e-06    3.449e-04
5.00    0.100    1.020e+07    2.455e-06    3.426e-04
5.00    0.200    9.783e+06    2.384e-06    3.358e-04
5.00    0.300    9.137e+06    2.273e-06    3.252e-04
5.00    0.400    8.333e+06    2.133e-06    3.116e-04
5.00    0.500    7.456e+06    1.979e-06    2.961e-04
5.00    0.600    6.603e+06    1.824e-06    2.803e-04
5.00    0.700    5.860e+06    1.686e-06    2.658e-04
5.00    0.800    5.294e+06    1.576e-06    2.541e-04
5.00    0.900    4.944e+06    1.505e-06    2.465e-04
5.00    1.000    4.825e+06    1.481e-06    2.438e-04

ncall =   831
```

```
# u1xx, u2xx, u3xx
  u1xx=dss044(xl,xu,nx,u1,u1x,nl,nu);
  u2xx=dss044(xl,xu,nx,u2,u2x,nl,nu);
  u3xx=dss044(xl,xu,nx,u3,u3x,nl,nu);
```

changed to

```
#
# u1x, u2x, u3x
  u1x=dss006(xl,xu,nx,u1);
  u2x=dss006(xl,xu,nx,u2);
  u3x=dss006(xl,xu,nx,u3);
                .
                .
                .
#
# u1xx, u2xx, u3xx
  u1xx=dss046(xl,xu,nx,u1,u1x,nl,nu);
  u2xx=dss046(xl,xu,nx,u2,u2x,nl,nu);
  u3xx=dss046(xl,xu,nx,u3,u3x,nl,nu);
```

Also, two `source` statements in Listing 2.4 have to be changed to access `dss006,dss046`.

Abbreviated output reflecting these changes is given as follows.

```
 dss004, dss044

    t        x      u1(x,t)      u2(x,t)      u3(x,t)
 5.00    0.000    1.034e+07    2.480e-06    3.449e-04
 5.00    0.100    1.020e+07    2.455e-06    3.426e-04
 5.00    0.200    9.783e+06    2.384e-06    3.358e-04
 5.00    0.300    9.137e+06    2.273e-06    3.252e-04
 5.00    0.400    8.333e+06    2.133e-06    3.116e-04
 5.00    0.500    7.456e+06    1.979e-06    2.961e-04
 5.00    0.600    6.603e+06    1.824e-06    2.803e-04
 5.00    0.700    5.860e+06    1.686e-06    2.658e-04
 5.00    0.800    5.294e+06    1.576e-06    2.541e-04
 5.00    0.900    4.944e+06    1.505e-06    2.465e-04
 5.00    1.000    4.825e+06    1.481e-06    2.438e-04

 ncall =   831
```

```
dss006, dss046

    t        x      u1(x,t)      u2(x,t)      u3(x,t)
 5.00    0.000    1.034e+07    2.480e-06    3.449e-04
 5.00    0.100    1.020e+07    2.455e-06    3.426e-04
 5.00    0.200    9.783e+06    2.384e-06    3.358e-04
 5.00    0.300    9.137e+06    2.273e-06    3.252e-04
 5.00    0.400    8.333e+06    2.133e-06    3.116e-04
 5.00    0.500    7.456e+06    1.979e-06    2.961e-04
 5.00    0.600    6.603e+06    1.824e-06    2.803e-04
 5.00    0.700    5.860e+06    1.686e-06    2.658e-04
 5.00    0.800    5.294e+06    1.576e-06    2.541e-04
 5.00    0.900    4.944e+06    1.505e-06    2.465e-04
 5.00    1.000    4.825e+06    1.481e-06    2.438e-04

 ncall =    831
```

Briefly, there is no perceptible change in the solution suggesting that the fourth-order approximations of `dss004,dss044` provided acceptable solution accuracy. This procedure of changing the order of the MOL approximations is termed *p refinement* because in the numerical analysis literature, the approximation order is often designated with p. For `dss004,dss044`, $p = 4$, whereas for `dss006,dss046`, $p = 6$.

2.4 Conclusions

In conclusion, the apparent accuracy of the numerical solution is due in part to a relatively smooth problem, because eqs. (2.6) have diffusion terms that tend to smooth any rapid changes in x and the Gaussian IC of eqs. (2.7) is smooth. For more stringent problems, this level of accuracy might not be as easily achieved. In other words, each new problem should be investigated numerically, with careful documentation of the apparent accuracy.

This concludes the discussion of the pattern formation models of eqs. (2.2) to (2.8). The 2-PDE and 3-PDE models would be difficult to investigate analytically, but computation of the numerical solutions was straightforward.

References

[1] Keller, E.F., and L.A. Segel (1971), Traveling bands of chemotactic bacteria: a theoretical analysis, *J. Theor. Biol.*, **30**, 235–248.

[2] Murray, J.D. (2003), *Mathematical Biology, II: Spatial Models and Biomedical Applications*, 3rd edition, Springer-Verlag, Berlin, Heidelberg.

CHAPTER 3

Belousov–Zhabotinskii Reaction System

3.1 Introduction

The PDE model discussed in this chapter pertains to the Belousov–Zhabotinskii (BZ) reaction system ([1], pp 35–36), which exhibits various types of dynamic behavior including oscillations and traveling waves. The intention is to demonstrate the numerical integration of a 2-PDE model for the BZ system including a special case for which one of the PDEs is the Fisher–Kolmogoroff equation. The numerical solutions are examined in some detail to discern when they exhibit traveling wave properties (as discussed in Chapter 1) and when they exhibit moving front properties that are not traveling waves.

3.2 The Belousov–Zhabotinskii Reaction System

The BZ reaction system is

$$BrO_3^- + Br^- \xrightarrow{k_1} HBrO_2 + HOBr \tag{3.1a}$$

$$HBrO_2 + Br^- \xrightarrow{k_2} 2HOBr \tag{3.1b}$$

$$BrO_3^- + HBrO_2 \xrightarrow{k_3} 2HBrO_2 \tag{3.1c}$$

$$2HBrO_2 \xrightarrow{k_4} BrO_3^- + HOBr \tag{3.1d}$$

Differential Equation Analysis in Biomedical Science and Engineering: Partial Differential Equation Applications with R, First Edition. William E. Schiesser.

The concentrations of the various chemical species in eqs. (3.1) are represented mathematically by the following variable names.

Equation variable	Chemical variable
a	BrO_3^-
p	HOBr
u_1	$HBrO_2$
u_2	Br^-

u_1, u_2 are the PDE dependent variables of interest in the subsequent (MOL) analysis.

Mass balances for u_1, u_2 are expressed as the following 1D reaction-diffusion PDEs.

$$\frac{\partial u_1}{\partial t} = D_1 \frac{\partial^2 u_1}{\partial x^2} + k_1 a u_2 - k_2 u_1 u_2 + k_3 a u_1 - k_4 u_1^2 \tag{3.2a}$$

$$\frac{\partial u_2}{\partial t} = D_2 \frac{\partial^2 u_2}{\partial x^2} - k_1 a u_2 - k_2 u_1 u_2 \tag{3.2b}$$

where x and t are space and time, respectively. The RHS diffusion terms are extensions of Fick's second law with diffusivities D_1, D_2.

The RHS reaction rate terms are based on mass action kinetics, with rate constants k_1, k_2, k_3, k_4. For example, in eq. (3.2a), the rate of reaction (3.1a) is expressed as

$$\text{rate of reaction} = k_1 a u_2$$

Note that the rate is proportional to the product of the concentrations of the reactants, a and u_2, which is the basic idea of mass action kinetics. The other reaction rates involving k_2, k_3, k_4 follow in a similar way from the concentrations of the reactants (if the reactions were reversible, the reaction rates would also include the concentrations of the products). Note that reaction rates of this form go to zero whenever the concentration of one or more reactants goes to zero as expected.

After the definition of dimensionless variables and the deletion of some terms through an order of magnitude analysis, the final 2-PDE system is ([1], eqs. (1.85))

$$\frac{\partial u_1}{\partial t} = \frac{\partial^2 u_1}{\partial x^2} + u_1(1 - u_1 - ru_2) \tag{3.3a}$$

$$\frac{\partial u_2}{\partial t} = \frac{\partial^2 u_2}{\partial x^2} - bu_1u_2 \tag{3.3b}$$

where r, b are positive constants of $O(1)$ (of order one). Eqs. (3.3) are the 2-PDE system to be integrated numerically.

Eqs. (3.3) each require one initial condition (IC) and two boundary conditions (BCs).

$$u_1(x, t = 0) = f_1(x);\ u_2(x, t = 0) = f_2(x) \tag{3.4a,b}$$

$$\frac{\partial u_1(x \to \infty, t)}{\partial x} = \frac{\partial u_1(x \to -\infty, t)}{\partial x} = 0 \tag{3.5a,b}$$

$$\frac{\partial u_2(x \to \infty, t)}{\partial x} = \frac{\partial u_2(x \to -\infty, t)}{\partial x} = 0 \tag{3.5c,d}$$

The requirement in applying BCs (3.5) is to select an interval or range in x that is sufficiently large to be essentially $\pm\infty$. The selection of the bounding values of x to satisfy this requirement is confirmed when the numerical solutions are examined.

$f_1(x), f_2(x)$ are taken as unit step functions in the subsequent programming. Thus, the solutions are a response to an initial discontinuity. This form of initial value problem is generally termed a *Riemann problem*. As we shall observe, the numerical solutions are smooth even with this discontinuity, which is a consequence of the diffusion based on $\partial^2 u_1/\partial x^2, \partial^2 u_2/\partial x^2$. The combination of a first-order derivative in t, that is, $\partial u_1/\partial t, \partial u_2/\partial t$, and the second-order derivative in x is termed a *parabolic PDE*, which generally smooths discontinuities. Hyperbolic PDEs, a second major class of time-dependent PDEs, propagate discontinuities and are therefore generally more difficult to integrate numerically (to accurately capture discontinuities).

The third major class of PDEs, elliptic, does not have derivatives with respect to an initial value variable (t) so that integration (of elliptic PDEs) generally requires a different class of numerical algorithms. Alternatively, an elliptic PDE can be converted to a parabolic PDE by adding a derivative in an initial value variable and then integrating the parabolic PDE until the initial value derivative effectively goes to zero; the resulting solution is for the elliptic PDE.

We now consider the MOL solution of eqs. (3.3)–(3.5).

3.2.1 ODE Routine

An ODE routine for eqs. (3.3) and (3.5) is in Listing 3.1.

```
  bz_1=function(t,u,parms){
#
# Function bz_1 computes the t derivative vector
# of the u1,u2 vectors
#
# One vector to two vectors
  u1=rep(0,nx);u2=rep(0,nx);
  for(i in 1:nx){
    u1[i]=u[i];
    u2[i]=u[i+nx];
  }
#
# u1x, u2x
  u1x=dss004(xl,xu,nx,u1);
  u2x=dss004(xl,xu,nx,u2);
#
# Boundary conditions
  u1x[1]=0;u1x[nx]=0;
  u2x[1]=0;u2x[nx]=0;
  nl=2;nu=2;
#
# u1xx, u2xx
  u1xx=dss044(xl,xu,nx,u1,u1x,nl,nu);
  u2xx=dss044(xl,xu,nx,u2,u2x,nl,nu);
#
# PDEs
```

```
  u1t=rep(0,nx);u2t=rep(0,nx);
  for(i in 1:nx){
    u1t[i]=u1xx[i]+u1[i]*(1-u1[i]-r*u2[i]);
    u2t[i]=u2xx[i]-b*u1[i]*u2[i];
  }
#
# Two vectors to one vector
  ut=rep(0,2*nx);
  for(i in 1:nx){
    ut[i]   =u1t[i];
    ut[i+nx]=u2t[i];
  }
#
# Increment calls to bz_1
  ncall <<- ncall+1;
#
# Return derivative vector
  return(list(c(ut)));
}
```

Listing 3.1 ODE routine `bz_1` for the MOL analysis of eqs. (3.3), (3.5).

We can note the following details about Listing 3.1.

- The function is defined.

  ```
    bz_1=function(t,u,parms){
  #
  # Function bz_1 computes the t derivative vector
  # of the u1,u2 vectors
  ```

  Concerning the RHS input arguments, (1) `t` is the current value of the independent variable t in eqs. (3.3), which can be used for the programming of functions of t, (2) `u` is a vector of dependent variables of length `2*nx=2*51=102` (`nx`, the number of points in x, is defined numerically in the main program to follow), and (3) `parms` that can be used to pass parameter values to `bz_1` is unused. The format of the three arguments (type and order) is required by the ODE integrator `lsodes`.

- The dependent variable vector u is placed in two vectors, u1,u2, to facilitate the programming of eqs. (3.3).

```
#
# One vector to two vectors
  u1=rep(0,nx);u2=rep(0,nx);
  for(i in 1:nx){
    u1[i]=u[i];
    u2[i]=u[i+nx];
  }
```

- The derivatives $\partial u_1/\partial x, \partial u_2/\partial x$ are computed by the library differentiation routine dss004. The boundary values of x, xl,xu, are defined numerically in the main program that follows.

```
#
# u1x, u2x
  u1x=dss004(xl,xu,nx,u1);
  u2x=dss004(xl,xu,nx,u2);
```

- BCs (3.5) are programmed, including the specification of the Neumann conditions (nl=2,nu=2).

```
#
# Boundary conditions
  u1x[1]=0;u1x[nx]=0;
  u2x[1]=0;u2x[nx]=0;
  nl=2;nu=2;
```

- The second derivatives $\partial^2 u_1/\partial x^2, \partial^2 u_2/\partial x^2$ are computed by dss044. Note that the BC first derivatives, u1x[1],u2x[1],u1[nx],u2[nx], are inputs to dss044.

```
#
# u1xx, u2xx
  u1xx=dss044(xl,xu,nx,u1,u1x,nl,nu);
  u2xx=dss044(xl,xu,nx,u2,u2x,nl,nu);
```

- Eqs. (3.3) are programmed in a for with index i. The similarity of this code with the equations, and the ease of including nonlinearities, for example, -b*u1[i]*u2[i], illustrates two of the principal features of the numerical approach.

```
#
# PDEs
  u1t=rep(0,nx);u2t=rep(0,nx);
  for(i in 1:nx){
    u1t[i]=u1xx[i]+u1[i]*(1-u1[i]-r*u2[i]);
    u2t[i]=u2xx[i]-b*u1[i]*u2[i];
  }
```

- The two derivative vectors `u1t,u2t` are placed in a single vector `ut` to be returned to the ODE integrator `lsodes`.

```
#
# Two vectors to one vector
  ut=rep(0,2*nx);
  for(i in 1:nx){
    ut[i]   =u1t[i];
    ut[i+nx]=u2t[i];
  }
```

- The counter for the calls to `bz_1` is incremented and returned to the main program with `<<-`.

```
#
# Increment calls to bz_1
  ncall <<- ncall+1;
```

  The final value of `ncall` at the completion of the solution is then displayed from the main program.
- The derivative vector `ut` is returned as a list (rather than as a numerical vector, a requirement of the R ODE integrators).

```
#
# Return derivative vector
  return(list(c(ut)));
}
```

  The final `}` concludes `bz_1`.

The programming in `bz_1` is for eqs. (3.3) and (3.5). All that remains is the programming of the ICs, eqs. (3.4), and the numerical specification of the model parameters, which is done in Section 3.2.2.

3.2.2 Main Program

Listing 3.2 parallels that of the previous main programs, for example, Listings 1.1 and 2.2.

```
#
# Access ODE integrator
  library("deSolve");
#
# Access functions for numerical solutions
  setwd("c:/R/bme_pde/chap3");
  source("bz_1.R");
  source("dss004.R");
  source("dss044.R");
#
# Level of output
#
#   ip = 1 - graphical (plotted) solutions
#            (u1(x,t), u2(x,t)) only
#
#   ip = 2 - numerical and graphical solutions
#
  ip=2;
#
# PDE coupling
#
#   ncase = 1 - two PDEs are uncoupled; first PDE (u1(x,t))
#               is the Fisher-Kolmogoroff equation
#
#   ncase = 2 - Belousov-Zhabotinskii reaction PDEs
#
# Grid (in x)
  nx=51;xl=-30;xu=20;
  xg=seq(from=xl,to=xu,by=(xu-xl)/(nx-1));
#
# Parameters, ICs
  ncase=1;
  if(ncase==1){
    b=1.25;r=0;
    nout=6;
```

```
    tout=seq(from=0,to=10,by=2);
  }
  if(ncase==2){
    b=1.25;r=10;
    nout=6;
    tout=seq(from=0,to=25,by=5);
  }
#
# Display parameters
  cat(sprintf(
    "\n\n  r = %5.2f  b = %6.3f\n",r,b));
#
# Initial condition
  u0=rep(0,2*nx);u10=rep(0,nx);u20=rep(0,nx);
  for(i in 1:nx){
#
#   Unit step at x = 0
    if(i<=25){
      u10[i]=0;u20[i]=1;
    }else if(i>=27){
      u10[i]=1;u20[i]=0;
    }else if(i==26){
      u10[i]=0.5;u20[i]=0.5;
    }
    u0[i]   =u10[i];
    u0[i+nx]=u20[i];
  }
  t=0;
  ncall=0;
#
# ODE integration
  out=lsodes(y=u0,times=tout,func=bz_1,parms=NULL)
  nrow(out)
  ncol(out)
#
# Arrays for plotting numerical solution
  u1_plot=matrix(0,nrow=nx,ncol=nout);
  u2_plot=matrix(0,nrow=nx,ncol=nout);
  for(it in 1:nout){
```

```
    for(ix in 1:nx){
       u1_plot[ix,it]=out[it,ix+1];
       u2_plot[ix,it]=out[it,ix+1+nx];
    }
  }
#
# Display numerical solution
  if(ip==2){
    for(it in 1:nout){
      cat(sprintf("\n\n     t      x   u1(x,t)
         u2(x,t)"));
      for(ix in 1:nx){
        cat(sprintf("\n%6.1f%7.1f%10.3f%10.3f",
          tout[it],xg[ix],u1_plot[ix,it],u2_plot
             [ix,it]));
      }
    }
  }
#
# Calls to ODE routine
  cat(sprintf("\n\n ncall = %5d\n\n",ncall));
#
# Plot u1, u2 numerical solutions
  if(ncase==1){
  par(mfrow=c(1,1));
  matplot(x=xg,y=u1_plot,type="l",xlab="x",
          ylab="u1(x,t), t=0,2,...,10",xlim=c(xl,xu),
             lty=1,main="u1(x,t); t=0,2,...,10;",lwd=2);
  par(mfrow=c(1,1));
  matplot(x=xg,y=u2_plot,type="l",xlab="x",
          ylab="u2(x,t), t=0,2,...,10",xlim=c(xl,xu),
             lty=1,main="u2(x,t); t=0,2,...,10;",lwd=2);
  }
  if(ncase==2){
  par(mfrow=c(1,1));
  matplot(x=xg,y=u1_plot,type="l",xlab="x",
          ylab="u1(x,t), t=0,5,...,25",xlim=c(xl,xu),
             lty=1,main="u1(x,t); t=0,5,...,25;",lwd=2);
  par(mfrow=c(1,1));
  matplot(x=xg,y=u2_plot,type="l",xlab="x",
          ylab="u2(x,t), t=0,5,...,25",xlim=c(xl,xu),
```

```
           lty=1,main="u2(x,t); t=0,5,...,25;",lwd=2);
}
```

Listing 3.2 Main program for the MOL analysis of eqs. (3.3)–(3.5).

We can note the following details about Listing 3.2.

- The R ODE library `deSolve` (with `lsodes`) and the ODE routine `bz_1` of Listing 3.1 are accessed.

```
#
# Access ODE integrator
  library("deSolve");
#
# Access functions for numerical solutions
  setwd("c:/R/bme_pde/chap3");
  source("bz_1.R");
  source("dss004.R");
  source("dss044.R");
```

- The level of output is specified with `ip`.

```
#
# PDE coupling
#
#   ncase = 1 - two PDEs are uncoupled; first PDE
#               (u1(x,t)) is the Fisher-Kolmogoroff
#               equation
#
#   ncase = 2 - Belousov-Zhabotinskii reaction PDEs
#
  ip=2;
```

- The range in x is defined.

```
#
# Grid (in x)
  nx=51;xl=-30;xu=20;
  xg=seq(from=xl,to=xu,by=(xu-xl)/(nx-1));
```

There are 51 points in x over the interval $-30 \le x \le 20$. The interval for $x < 0$ is larger because of the right to left movement of the traveling wave (for ncase=1) and moving front (for ncase=2) solutions.

- The interval in t is different for ncase=1,2. In particular, for ncase=1 and $r = 0$, eq. (3.3a) is uncoupled from eq. (3.3b) (eq. (3.3a) is then the Fisher–Kolmogoroff equation as explained subsequently), and the corresponding traveling wave solution moves right to left at a higher velocity so that a shorter interval in t is used.

```
#
# Parameters, ICs
  ncase=1;
  if(ncase==1){
    b=1.25;r=0;
    nout=6;
    tout=seq(from=0,to=10,by=2);
  }
  if(ncase==2){
    b=1.25;r=10;
    nout=6;
    tout=seq(from=0,to=25,by=5);
  }
```

For ncase=2 and $r \neq 0$ ($r > 0$), the slower movement of the solution front requires a larger interval in t for resolution of the solution. These features are demonstrated in the graphical output to follow.

- The parameters r, b in eqs. (3.3) are displayed.

```
#
# Display parameters
  cat(sprintf(
    "\n\n  r = %5.2f  b = %6.3f\n",r,b));
```

- The ICs of eqs. (3.4) are programmed as unit steps with a for in i. Since the grid in x has nx=51 points, the midpoint is at i=26. To the left of this point (i<26), $u_1(x, t = 0) = 0, u_2(x, t = 0) = 1$. To the right of i=26 (i>26), $u_1(x, t = 0) = 1, u_2(x, t = 0) = 0$.

At i=26, the mid values $u_1(x, t = 0) = u_2(x, t = 0) = 0.5$ are used.

```
#
# Initial condition
  u0=rep(0,2*nx);u10=rep(0,nx);u20=rep(0,nx);
  for(i in 1:nx){
#
#   Unit step
    if(i<=25){
      u10[i]=0;u20[i]=1;
    }else if(i>=27){
      u10[i]=1;u20[i]=0;
    }else if(i==26){
      u10[i]=0.5;u20[i]=0.5;
    }
    u0[i]    =u10[i];
    u0[i+nx]=u20[i];
  }
  ncall=0;
```

After definition of the unit steps, the two ICs are placed in a single IC vector `u0` as an input to `lsodes`. Finally, the number of calls to `bz_1` is initialized.

- The `2*51` = 102 ODEs are integrated by `lsodes`. Note the RHS inputs: (1) `y` as the IC vector (the length of `u0`, `102`, informs `lsodes` of the number of ODEs to be integrated); (2) `times` as the vector of output values of t, `tout`, defined previously; (3) `func` for the ODE routine `bz_1`; and (4) `parms` for parameters to be passed to `bz_1` (unused). `y,times,func,parms` are reserved names.

```
#
# ODE integration
  out=lsodes(y=u0,times=tout,func=bz_1,parms=NULL)
  nrow(out)
  ncol(out)
```

The numerical solution is returned in the 2D array `out`. The dimensions of `out` are displayed with the R `nrow,ncol` utilities.

- The two PDE solutions, $u_1(x,t), u_2(x,t)$, are placed in two 2D arrays, u1_plot,u2_plot, for subsequent plotting. The subscripts [ix,it] specify the variation in the solutions with respect to x and t, respectively.

```
#
# Arrays for plotting numerical solution
  u1_plot=matrix(0,nrow=nx,ncol=nout);
  u2_plot=matrix(0,nrow=nx,ncol=nout);
  for(it in 1:nout){
    for(ix in 1:nx){
       u1_plot[ix,it]=out[it,ix+1];
       u2_plot[ix,it]=out[it,ix+1+nx];
    }
  }
```

Note the offset in the second subscript of 1, for example, ix+1, because out[it,1] is reserved for the value of t corresponding to each output point it (rather than for an ODE dependent variable). Thus, the dimensions of out are out[nout,2*nx+1] =out[6,2*51+1]=out[6,103], which are confirmed with the above nrow,ncol statements.

- For ip=2, the solutions of eqs. (3.3) are displayed as a function of x and t.

```
#
# Display numerical solution
  if(ip==2){
    for(it in 1:nout){
      cat(sprintf("\n\n     t      x   u1(x,t)
         u2(x,t)"));
      for(ix in 1:nx){
        cat(sprintf("\n%6.1f%7.1f%10.3f%10.3f",
          tout[it],xg[ix],u1_plot[ix,it],u2_
             plot[ix,it]));
      }
    }
  }
```

The inner for with index ix gives the variation of the solutions with x, and the outer for with index it gives the variation with t.

- The number of calls to bz_1 at the end of the solution is displayed as a measure of the effort required to compute the solution.

```
#
# Calls to ODE routine
  cat(sprintf("\n\n ncall = %5d\n\n",ncall));
```

- For ncase=1, the solutions $u_1(x,t), u_2(x,t)$ are plotted over the interval $0 \leq t \leq 10$. The par(mfrow=c(1,1)) specifies one plot for each dependent variable.

```
#
# Plot u1, u2 numerical solutions
  if(ncase==1){
  par(mfrow=c(1,1));
  matplot(x=xg,y=u1_plot,type="l",xlab="x",
          ylab="u1(x,t), t=0,2,...,10",xlim=c(xl,xu),
             lty=1,main="u1(x,t); t=0,2,...,10;",
                lwd=2);
  par(mfrow=c(1,1));
  matplot(x=xg,y=u2_plot,type="l",xlab="x",
          ylab="u2(x,t), t=0,2,...,10",xlim=c(xl,xu),
             lty=1,main="u2(x,t); t=0,2,...,10;",
                lwd=2);
  }
```

Similarly, for ncase=2, the solutions are plotted over the interval $0 \leq t \leq 25$,

This completes the programming of eqs. (3.3)–(3.5). The output from Listings 3.1 and 3.2 is now considered for ncase=1,2.

3.2.3 Model Output

For ncase=1, the abbreviated output is given in Table 3.1.
We can note the following details about this output.

- At $t = 0$, the unit steps in u1,u2 occur at x=-5 as discussed previously.

TABLE 3.1 Abbreviated output from Listing 3.2 for `ncase=1`.

```
r =  0.00  b =  1.250

> nrow(out)
[1] 6
> ncol(out)
[1] 103

   t       x   u1(x,t)   u2(x,t)
 0.0   -30.0     0.000     1.000
 0.0   -29.0     0.000     1.000
 0.0   -28.0     0.000     1.000
 0.0   -27.0     0.000     1.000
 0.0   -26.0     0.000     1.000
           .       .
           .       .
           .       .
Output for x = -25 to -8 removed
           .       .
           .       .
           .       .
 0.0    -7.0     0.000     1.000
 0.0    -6.0     0.000     1.000
 0.0    -5.0     0.500     0.500
 0.0    -4.0     1.000     0.000
 0.0    -3.0     1.000     0.000
           .       .
           .       .
           .       .
Output for x = -2 to 15 removed
           .       .
           .       .
           .       .
 0.0    16.0     1.000     0.000
 0.0    17.0     1.000     0.000
 0.0    18.0     1.000     0.000
 0.0    19.0     1.000     0.000
```

TABLE 3.1 (*Continued*)

```
  0.0   20.0     1.000     0.000
           .       .
           .       .
           .       .
 Output for t = 2,4,6,8 removed
           .       .
           .       .
           .       .
    t      x   u1(x,t)   u2(x,t)
 10.0  -30.0     0.000     1.000
 10.0  -29.0     0.000     0.999
 10.0  -28.0     0.001     0.998
 10.0  -27.0     0.004     0.995
 10.0  -26.0     0.010     0.987
 10.0  -25.0     0.025     0.969
 10.0  -24.0     0.056     0.931
 10.0  -23.0     0.112     0.864
 10.0  -22.0     0.198     0.762
 10.0  -21.0     0.315     0.629
 10.0  -20.0     0.447     0.484
 10.0  -19.0     0.579     0.348
 10.0  -18.0     0.695     0.236
 10.0  -17.0     0.788     0.153
 10.0  -16.0     0.856     0.096
 10.0  -15.0     0.905     0.058
 10.0  -14.0     0.938     0.035
 10.0  -13.0     0.960     0.021
 10.0  -12.0     0.975     0.012
 10.0  -11.0     0.984     0.007
 10.0  -10.0     0.990     0.004
           .       .
           .       .
           .       .
 Output for x = -8 to 15 removed
           .       .
           .       .
           .       .
```

(*continued*)

TABLE 3.1 *(Continued)*

```
10.0    16.0      1.000      0.000
10.0    17.0      1.000      0.000
10.0    18.0      1.000      0.000
10.0    19.0      1.000      0.000
10.0    20.0      1.000      0.000

ncall =  227
```

- These steps move right to left with some smoothing (note the solutions at $t = 10$ and around $x = -20$).
- BCs (3.5) are satisfied (the slopes or derivatives with respect to x appear to be zero at the boundaries $x = -30, 20$).
- The computational effort is modest with `ncall = 227`.

The solutions can be visualized in Figs. 3.1 and 3.2. In Fig. 3.1, $u_1(x,t)$ moves as a traveling wave. Specifically, as discussed in Chapter 1, the solution appears to be a function of the Lagrangian variable $z = x - ct$ where c is the velocity. Thus, since the curves correspond to constant intervals in t, that is, $t = 0, 2, 4, 6, 8, 10$, the curves are displaced in constant intervals of x. This property of a traveling wave solution (function of z only) is a well-known feature of the Fisher–Kolmogoroff equation (eq. (3.3a) with $r = 0$).

Similarly, $u_2(x,t)$ in Fig. 3.2 displays a solution that appears to be a traveling wave (note that eq. (3.3b) is coupled to eq. (3.3a) even with $r = 0$).

For `ncase=2`, the abbreviated output is given in Table 3.2. We can note the following details about this output.

- At $t = 0$, the unit steps in `u1,u2` occur at `x=-5` as discussed previously.
- The solutions for $t > 0$ are rather complicated. For example, $u_1(x,t)$ moves left to right, whereas $u_2(x,t)$ moves right to left.
- The computational effort is modest with `ncall = 266`.

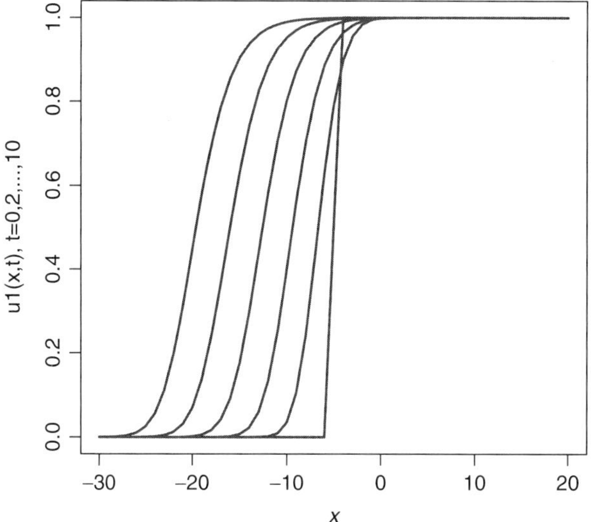

Figure 3.1 $u_1(x,t)$ versus x with t as a parameter, ncase=1.

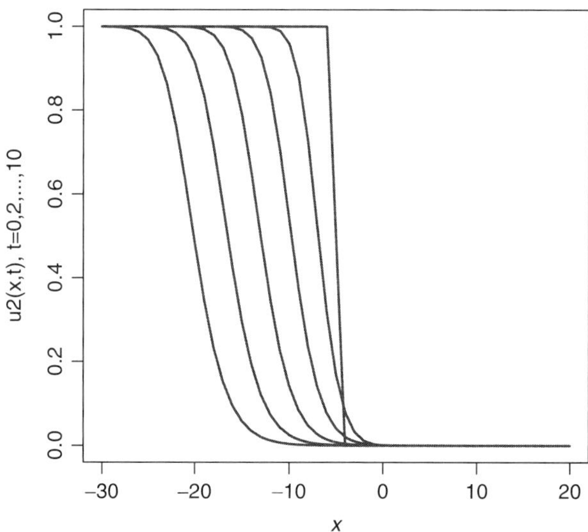

Figure 3.2 $u_2(x,t)$ versus x with t as a parameter, ncase=1.

TABLE 3.2 Abbreviated output from Listing 3.2 for `ncase=2`.

```
r = 10.00  b =  1.250

> nrow(out)
[1] 6
> ncol(out)
[1] 103

   t      x   u1(x,t)   u2(x,t)
 0.0  -30.0     0.000     1.000
 0.0  -29.0     0.000     1.000
 0.0  -28.0     0.000     1.000
 0.0  -27.0     0.000     1.000
 0.0  -26.0     0.000     1.000
          .       .
          .       .
          .       .
Output for x = -25 to -8 removed
          .       .
          .       .
          .       .
 0.0   -7.0     0.000     1.000
 0.0   -6.0     0.000     1.000
 0.0   -5.0     0.500     0.500
 0.0   -4.0     1.000     0.000
 0.0   -3.0     1.000     0.000
          .       .
          .       .
          .       .
Output for x = -2 to 15 removed
          .       .
          .       .
          .       .
 0.0   16.0     1.000     0.000
 0.0   17.0     1.000     0.000
 0.0   18.0     1.000     0.000
 0.0   19.0     1.000     0.000
 0.0   20.0     1.000     0.000
```

TABLE 3.2 (*Continued*)

```
          .       .
          .       .
          .       .
  Output for t = 5,10,15,20 removed
          .       .
          .       .
          .       .
     t       x    u1(x,t)    u2(x,t)
  25.0   -30.0      0.000      1.000
  25.0   -29.0      0.000      0.999
  25.0   -28.0     -0.000      0.999
  25.0   -27.0     -0.000      0.999
  25.0   -26.0      0.000      0.998
          .       .
          .       .
          .       .
  Output for x = -25 to -16 removed
          .       .
          .       .
          .       .
  25.0   -15.0     -0.000      0.901
  25.0   -14.0     -0.000      0.871
  25.0   -13.0     -0.000      0.835
  25.0   -12.0     -0.000      0.792
  25.0   -11.0     -0.000      0.741
  25.0   -10.0     -0.000      0.682
  25.0    -9.0      0.000      0.615
  25.0    -8.0      0.000      0.540
  25.0    -7.0      0.001      0.456
  25.0    -6.0      0.005      0.366
  25.0    -5.0      0.027      0.270
  25.0    -4.0      0.097      0.177
  25.0    -3.0      0.254      0.099
  25.0    -2.0      0.479      0.046
  25.0    -1.0      0.693      0.019
  25.0     0.0      0.842      0.007
  25.0     1.0      0.926      0.003
  25.0     2.0      0.967      0.001
```

(*continued*)

TABLE 3.2 (*Continued*)

```
                 .       .
                 .       .
                 .       .
 Output for x = 3 to 15 removed
                 .       .
                 .       .
                 .       .
 25.0    16.0      1.000      0.000
 25.0    17.0      1.000      0.000
 25.0    18.0      1.000      0.000
 25.0    19.0      1.000      0.000
 25.0    20.0      1.000      0.000

 ncall =   266
```

The solutions can be visualized in Figs. 3.3 and 3.4. In Fig. 3.3, $u_1(x,t)$ moves as a front (left to right) that appears to have a steady form (little change with t for $t > 0$). Thus, $u_1(x,t)$ appears to be not a traveling wave (function of z only).

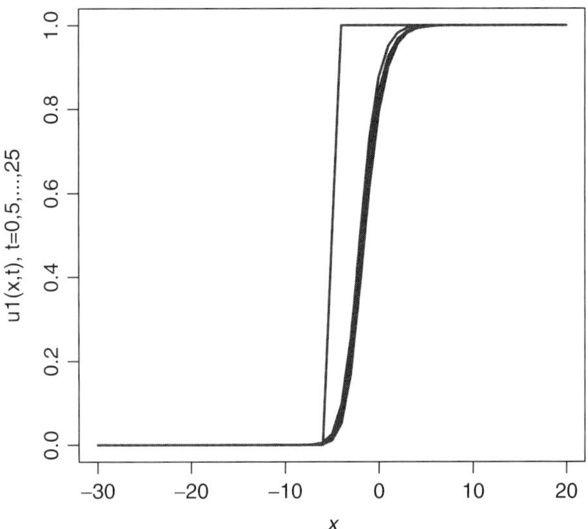

Figure 3.3 $u_1(x,t)$ versus x with t as a parameter, ncase=2.

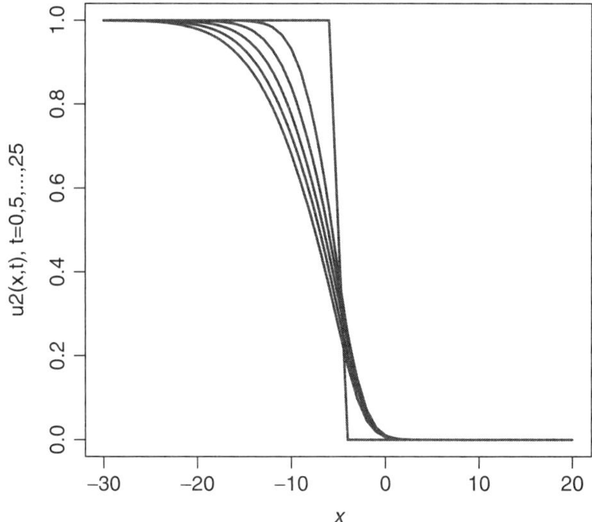

Figure 3.4 $u_2(x,t)$ versus x with t as a parameter, `ncase=2`.

$u_2(x,t)$ in Fig. 3.4 displays a solution that is a front moving right to left but appears to be not a traveling wave (with constant intervals in x and t).

In summary, the solutions $u_1(x,t), u_2(x,t)$ change form substantially with a change in only r from $r = 0$ (`ncase=1`) to $r = 10$ (`ncase=2`).

3.3 Conclusions

The numerical solution of eqs. (3.3)–(3.5) is straightforward and the effect of variations in the parameters, e.g., r, is easily investigated. To conclude this study, the accuracy of the solutions should be investigated, for example, by changing the number of points x (51 appears to be adequate) and the order of the numerical differentiation in x (`dss004,dss044` appear to be adequate). The results of this application of h and p refinement are not reported here to conserve space but can easily be carried out by the reader.

Reference

[1] Murray, J.D. (2003), *Mathematical Biology, II: Spatial Models and Biomedical Applications*, 3rd Edition, Springer-Verlag, Berlin, Heidelberg.

CHAPTER 4

Hodgkin–Huxley and Fitzhugh–Nagumo Models

4.1 Introduction

A mathematical model for excitable media, with application to neuron dynamics, was proposed by Fitzhugh [1] as a special case of an earlier model by Hodgkin and Huxley [3]. The Fitzhugh model is a 2×2 nonlinear ODE system (with just temporal effects) that was then extended by Nagumo [5] to include spatial effects in the form of Fickian diffusion. The resulting Fitzhugh-Nagumo 1D 1×1 (single) PDE model is the starting point for this chapter.

Since this model has been discussed extensively, e.g., [4], we focus here on the MOL computation of numerical solutions. Also, an analytical solution is available that is used to evaluate the numerical solution.

In this chapter, we consider the following topics.

- An introduction to the FHN PDE.
- Algorithms for the numerical solution of the FHN PDE.
- Computer routines for implementation of the numerical algorithms, including the implementation of a series of BCs.
- Traveling wave features of the FHN model with a comparison of the analytical and numerical solutions.

Differential Equation Analysis in Biomedical Science and Engineering: Partial Differential Equation Applications with R, First Edition. William E. Schiesser.

4.2 PDE Model

The FHN PDE is

$$\frac{\partial u}{\partial t} = D\frac{\partial^2 u}{\partial x^2} - u(1-u)(a-u) \tag{4.1a}$$

where a and D are arbitrary constants with $0 \le a \le 1$, $D > 0$. Note, in particular, the cubic nonlinearity in u.

The following traveling wave solution to eq. (4.1) ([2], pp 166–171; [6], p4) is used to evaluate the numerical solution

$$u(x,t) = \frac{1}{1+\exp\left[\dfrac{x}{\sqrt{2D}} + \left(a - \dfrac{1}{2}\right)t\right]} \tag{4.2a}$$

Eq. (4.2a) is used to specify the IC for eq. (4.1) at $t = 0$.

$$u(x,t=0) = \frac{1}{1+\exp\left[\dfrac{x}{\sqrt{2D}}\right]} \tag{4.1b}$$

Also, boundary conditions (BCs) for eq. (4.1a) discussed subsequently include Neumann BCs that require the derivative $\partial u(x,t)/\partial x$. This derivative from eq. (4.2a) is

$$\frac{\partial u(x,t)}{\partial x} = \frac{-\exp\left[\dfrac{x}{\sqrt{2D}} + \left(a-\dfrac{1}{2}\right)t\right]\dfrac{1}{\sqrt{2D}}}{\left\{1+\exp\left[\dfrac{x}{\sqrt{2D}} + \left(a-\dfrac{1}{2}\right)t\right]\right\}^2} \tag{4.2b}$$

We now consider the MOL solution of eqs. (4.1) with a series of BCs, including analytical BCs from eqs. (4.2).

4.3 MOL Routines

A main program and subordinate ODE routine for eqs. (4.1) and (4.2) are discussed in the following sections.

4.3.1 ODE Routine

An ODE routine for eqs. (4.1) and (4.2) is in Listing 4.1

```
  fhn_1=function(t,u,parms){
#
# Function fhn_1 computes the t derivative vector for the
# Fitzhugh-Nagumo equation
#
# Analytical Dirichlet BCs at x = 0,1
  if(ncase==1){
     u[1] =ua_1(xg[1] ,t);
     u[nx]=ua_1(xg[nx],t);
  }
#
# Constant Dirichlet BCs at x = 0,1
  if(ncase==2){
     u[1] =1;
     u[nx]=0;
  }
#
# ux
  ux=rep(0,nx);
  ux=dss004(xl,xu,nx,u);
#
# Analytical Neumann BCs at x=0,1
  if(ncase==3){
     ux[1] =uxa_1(xg[1] ,t);
     ux[nx]=uxa_1(xg[nx],t);
  }
#
# Homogeneous Neumann BCs at x=0,1
  if(ncase==4){
     ux[1] =0;
     ux[nx]=0;
  }
#
# No BCs at x=0,1
  if(ncase==5){
  }
#
# uxx
```

```
  uxx=rep(0,nx);
  uxx=dss004(xl,xu,nx,ux);
#
# PDE
  ut=rep(0,nx);
  if((ncase==1)||(ncase==2)){
    for(i in 2:(nx-1)){
      ut[i]=D*uxx[i]-u[i]*(1-u[i])*(a-u[i]);
    }
    ut[1]=0;
   ut[nx]=0;
  }
  if((ncase==3)||(ncase==4)||(ncase==5)){
    for(i in 1:nx){
      ut[i]=D*uxx[i]-u[i]*(1-u[i])*(a-u[i]);
    }
   }
#
# Increment calls to fhn_1
  ncall <<- ncall+1;
#
# Return derivative vector
  return(list(c(ut)));
  }
```

Listing 4.1 ODE routine `fhn_1` for eqs. (4.1) and (4.2).

We can note the following points about `fhn_1`.

- The function is defined, with the three input arguments required by the ODE integrator `lsodes`. `t` is the current value of t in eq. (4.1a), and `u` is a vector of values of $u(x,t)$ in eq. (4.1a). The length of `u` is `nx=101` with `nx` defined numerically in the main program discussed subsequently. `parms` for passing parameters to `fhn_1` is unused.

```
  fhn_1=function(t,u,parms){
#
# Function fhn_1 computes the t derivative vector for
# the Fitzhugh-Nagumo equation
```

- Five cases are programmed with `ncase=1,2,3,4,5` defined numerically in the main program and passed to `fhn_1`. For `ncase=1`, the Dirichlet BCs at $x = 0, 1$ are defined by the analytical solution of eq. (4.2a).

```
#
# Analytical Dirichlet BCs at x = 0,1
  if(ncase==1){
     u[1] =ua_1(xg[1] ,t);
     u[nx]=ua_1(xg[nx],t);
  }
```

  `ua_1` is a function for the analytical solution of eq. (4.2a) discussed subsequently. Note the use of `xg[1],xg[nx]` for the boundary values $x = 0, 1$. The grid in x, `xg`, is defined numerically in the main program (with `nx=101`); that is, `xg[1]=0,xg[2]=0.01,...,xg[nx]=1`. Also, the boundary values can change with t (the second argument of `ua_1`), but for this particular case, the boundary values do not change with t as indicated for `ncase=2` (next).

- For `ncase=2`, the Dirichlet BCs are specified as constant values.

```
#
# Constant Dirichlet BCs at x = 0,1
  if(ncase==2){
     u[1] =1;
     u[nx]=0;
  }
```

  This choice of the boundary values follows from the observation of the analytical solution at the boundaries (i.e., from the output for `ncase=1`). Setting the Dirichlet BCs at specific values is more typical in applications when an analytical solution is not available. Also, the use of constant boundary values presupposes the traveling wave solution (discussed next) does not reach the boundaries and thereby change the boundary values.

- The derivative $\partial u(x,t)/\partial x$ is computed by a call to the differentiation routine `dss004`. The previously defined boundary values, for example, $u(x = 0) = 1, u(x = 1, t) = 0$ for ncase=2, are used in the calculations in dss004 (through the fourth input argument). xl=0,xu=1 are defined numerically in the main program.

```
#
# ux
  ux=rep(0,nx);
  ux=dss004(xl,xu,nx,u);
```

- For ncase=3, Neumann BCs are used from eq. (4.2b).

```
#
# Analytical Neumann BCs at x=0,1
  if(ncase==3){
     ux[1] =uxa_1(xg[1] ,t);
     ux[nx]=uxa_1(xg[nx],t);
  }
```

uxa_1 is a function for the derivative $\partial u(x,a)/\partial x$ from eq. (4.2b). Note again the use of the boundary values xg[1],xg[nx]. Also, the derivatives in x, ux[1] and ux[nx], do not change with t as indicated in ncase=4 (next).

- For ncase=4, Neumann BCs are specified as homogeneous (zero).

```
#
# Homogeneous Neumann BCs at x=0,1
  if(ncase==4){
     ux[1] =0;
     ux[nx]=0;
  }
```

This choice of the homogeneous Neumann BCs follows from the observation of the analytical solution at the boundaries (i.e., from the output for ncase=1,3). Setting the Neumann BCs at specific values is more typical in applications when an analytical solution is not available, for example, to specify a no-flux (no-diffusion or insulated) BC. Also, the use of constant BCs presupposes the traveling wave solution does not reach the boundaries and thereby change the BCs.

- Since for `ncase=1,2,3,4,` the BCs actually have no effect on the solution (the traveling wave does not reach the boundaries), `ncase=5` corresponds to no BCs. That is, eq. (4.1a) constitutes an entirely initial value problem (and not an initial-boundary value problem). This situation with no BCs is somewhat unusual and results from the characteristics of this particular problem. More generally, a PDE nth order in the spatial independent variable (such as x) requires n BCs; for eq. (4.1a), $n = 2$.

```
#
# No BCs at x=0,1
  if(ncase==5){
  }
```

- The second derivative $\partial^2 u/\partial x^2$ is computed by differentiating the first derivative $\partial u/\partial x$, using so-called stagewise differentiation.

```
#
# uxx
  uxx=rep(0,nx);
  uxx=dss004(xl,xu,nx,ux);
```

- Eq. (4.1a) is programmed for Dirichlet BCs (`ncase=1,2`).

```
#
# PDE
  ut=rep(0,nx);
  if((ncase==1)||(ncase==2)){
    for(i in 2:(nx-1)){
      ut[i]=D*uxx[i]-u[i]*(1-u[i])*(a-u[i]);
    }
    ut[1]=0;
   ut[nx]=0;
  }
```

`||` is the `or` operator for scalars in R. Note that the ODEs at the boundaries in x are programmed with zero derivatives because the values of $u(x,t)$ at these two points are set by the (constant) BCs, that is, they are invariant with t. The close resemblance of eq. (4.1a) and the programming is clear.

- Eq. (4.1a) is programmed for Neumann BCs (ncase=3,4) and no BCs (ncase=5).

```
if((ncase==3)||(ncase==4)||(ncase==5)){
  for(i in 1:nx){
    ut[i]=D*uxx[i]-u[i]*(1-u[i])*(a-u[i]);
  }
 }
```

  nx ODEs are defined in the for because the boundary values of $u(x,t)$ can change with t.

- The number of calls to fhn_1 is incremented and returned to the main program with <<-.

```
#
# Increment calls to fhn_1
  ncall <<- ncall+1;
```

- The derivative vector ut is returned to lsodes as a R vector with c and then a list.

```
#
# Return derivative vector
  return(list(c(ut)));
  }
```

  The final } concludes fhn_1.

Functions ua_1 and uax_1 for the analytical solution of eq. (4.2a) and its derivative in x, eq. (4.2b), are in Listings 4.2a and 4.2b.

```
  ua_1=function(x,t){
#
# Function ua_1 computes the analytical solution for
# the Fitzhugh-Nagumo equation
#
```

```
  ua=1/(1+exp((1/2^0.5)*x/D^0.5+(a-1/2)*t));
  return(c(ua));
  }
```

Listing 4.2a ua_1 for eq. (4.2a).

```
  uxa_1=function(x,t){
#
# Function uxa_1 computes the x derivative of the
# analytical solution for the Fitzhugh-Nagumo equation
#
  expa=exp((1/(2*D)^0.5)*x+(a-1/2)*t);
  uxa=-expa*(1/(2*D)^0.5)/(1+expa)^2;
  return(c(uxa));
  }
```

Listing 4.2b uax_1 for eq. (4.2b).

These routines are essentially self-explanatory through comparison with eqs. (4.2). D and a are defined numerically in the following main program.

4.3.2 Main Program

The main program for eqs. (4.1) and (4.2) is listed next.

```
#
# Access ODE integrator
  library("deSolve");
#
# Access functions for analytical, numerical solutions
  setwd("c:/R/bme_pde/chap4");
  source("fhn_1.R");
  source("u0_1.R");
  source("ua_1.R");
  source("uxa_1.R");
  source("dss004.R");
#
# Level of output
#
#   ip = 1 - graphical (plotted) solutions
#            (u(x,t)) only
```

```
#
#   ip = 2 - numerical and graphical solutions
#
  ip=2;
#
# Alternative boundary conditions (BCs)
#
#   ncase = 1 - analytical Dirichlet BCs
#
#   ncase = 2 - constant Dirichlet BCs
#
#   ncase = 3 - analytical Neumann BCs
#
#   ncase = 4 - homogeneous Neumann BCs
#
#   ncase = 5 - no BCs
#
  ncase=1;
#
# Parameters
  a=1;D=1;
  cat(sprintf("\n\n a = %5.2f   D = %5.2f\n",a,D));
#
# Grid (in x)
  nx=101;xl=-60;xu=20;
  xg=seq(from=xl,to=xu,by=(xu-xl)/(nx-1));
#
# Independent variable for ODE integration
  nout=7;
  tout=seq(from=0,to=60,by=10);
#
# Initial condition (from analytical solution,t=0)
  u0=rep(0,nx);t0=0;
  u0=u0_1(t0);
  ncall=0;
#
# ODE integration
  out=lsodes(y=u0,times=tout,func=fhn_1,parms=NULL)
  nrow(out)
  ncol(out)
#
```

```
# Arrays for plotting numerical, analytical solutions
  u_plot=matrix(0,nrow=nx,ncol=nout);
 ua_plot=matrix(0,nrow=nx,ncol=nout);
 for(it in 1:nout){
   for(ix in 1:nx){
       u_plot[ix,it]=out[it,ix+1];
      ua_plot[ix,it]=ua_1(xg[ix],tout[it]);
   }
 }
#
# Display numerical solution
  if(ip==2){
    for(it in 1:nout){
      cat(sprintf("\n    t       x    u(x,t)   u_ex(x,t)
         u_err(x,t)\n"));
      for(ix in 1:nx){
        cat(sprintf("%5.1f%8.2f%10.5f%12.5f%13.6f\n",
           tout[it],xg[ix],
        u_plot[ix,it],ua_plot[ix,it],u_plot[ix,it]-ua_plot
           [ix,it]));
      }
    }
  }
#
# Calls to ODE routine
  cat(sprintf("\n\n ncall = %5d\n\n",ncall));
#
# Plot u numerical, analytical solution
  par(mfrow=c(1,1));
  matplot(x=xg,y=u_plot,type="l",xlab="x",ylab="u1(x,t),
     t=0,10,...,60",xlim=c(xl,xu),lty=1,main="u(x,t);
        solid - num, points - anal; t=0,10,...,60;",lwd=2);
  matpoints(x=xg,y=ua_plot,xlim=c(xl,xu),col="black",
     lwd=2)
```

Listing 4.3 Main program for eqs. (4.1) and (4.2).

We can note the following details about this main program.

- The ODE integrator library `deSolve` and a series of routines are accessed. In particular, the ODE routine `fhn_1` of Listing 4.1

is included. u0_1 is a routine to define the IC of eq. (4.1b) as discussed below.

```
#
# Access ODE integrator
  library("deSolve");
#
# Access functions for analytical, numerical solutions
  setwd("c:/R/bme_pde/chap4");
  source("fhn_1.R");
  source("u0_1.R");
  source("ua_1.R");
  source("uxa_1.R");
  source("dss004.R");
```

Note the use of the forward slash (/) rather than the usual backslash (\) in the setwd.

- The level of output is selected with ip.

```
#
# Level of output
#
#   ip = 1 - graphical (plotted) solutions
#            (u(x,t)) only
#
#   ip = 2 - numerical and graphical solutions
#
  ip=2;
```

- The five cases for ncase=1,2,3,4,5 used in fhn_1 are delineated.

```
#
# Alternative boundary conditions (BCs)
#
#   ncase = 1 - analytical Dirichlet BCs
#
#   ncase = 2 - constant Dirichlet BCs
#
#   ncase = 3 - analytical Neumann BCs
#
```

```
#   ncase = 4 - homogeneous Neumann BCs
#
#   ncase = 5 - no BCs
#
  ncase=1;
```

- The parameters a, D in eqs. (4.1) and (4.2) are specified.

```
#
# Parameters
  a=1;D=1;
  cat(sprintf("\n\n a = %5.2f   D = %5.2f\n",a,D));
```

Specifically, $a = 1$ defines the traveling wave velocity as discussed subsequently, and $D = 1$ defines the degree of smoothing of the traveling wave front.

- The grid in x is defined with $nx = 101$ points for the interval $-60 \leq x \leq 20$ with the `seq`. Thus, the values of x with spacing 0.8 are $x = -60, -59.2, \ldots, 20$.

```
#
# Grid (in x)
  nx=101;xl=-60;xu=20;
  xg=seq(from=xl,to=xu,by=(xu-xl)/(nx-1));
```

The interval in x is not symmetric with respect to $x = 0$ because the traveling waves move right to left ($a = 1$ corresponds to a negative velocity as explained below).

- The interval in t is $0 \leq t \leq 60$ with 7 output values for the numerical and analytical solutions.

```
#
# Independent variable for ODE integration
  nout=7;
  tout=seq(from=0,to=60,by=10);
```

That is, the solution is displayed at $t = 0, 10, \ldots, 60$.

- The IC of eq. (4.1b) is defined by a call to a function `u0_1` (discussed next).

```
#
# Initial condition (from analytical solution,t=0)
  u0=rep(0,nx);t0=0;
  u0=u0_1(t0);
  ncall=0;
```

u0_1 calls ua_1 of Listing 4.2a for $t = 0$. Also, the counter for the calls to fhn_1 is initialized.

- The 101 MOL ODEs are integrated by lsodes. Note the use of the IC vector, u0, the vector of output values of t, tout, and the use of fhn_1, as expected. The length of tout (101) informs lsodes of the number of ODEs to be integrated.

```
#
# ODE integration
  out=lsodes(y=u0,times=tout,func=fhn_1,parms=NULL)
  nrow(out)
  ncol(out)
```

y,times,func,parms are reserved names of lsodes. parms for passing parameters to fhn_1 is unused. The dimensions of the output solution array out are out[7,102] as displayed by nrow,ncol (in the output that follows); the column dimension of out is 102 rather than 101 because the second dimension includes t as well as the 101 values of u (of eq. (4.1a)).

- Arrays are defined for the numerical and analytical solutions. The numerical solution is provided by array out from lsodes (with the offset ix+1 because t is also included in out), and the analytical solution is provided through calls to ua_1 of Listing 4.2a.

```
#
# Arrays for plotting numerical, analytical solutions
   u_plot=matrix(0,nrow=nx,ncol=nout);
  ua_plot=matrix(0,nrow=nx,ncol=nout);
  for(it in 1:nout){
    for(ix in 1:nx){
        u_plot[ix,it]=out[it,ix+1];
       ua_plot[ix,it]=ua_1(xg[ix],tout[it]);
```

```
    }
  }
```

The for in it steps through the seven values of t and the for in ix steps through the 101 values of x to numerically define $u(x,t)$ in eq. (4.1a).

- The analytical and numerical solutions, and their difference (which is the exact error in the numerical solution), are displayed for ip=2.

```
#
# Display numerical solution
  if(ip==2){
    for(it in 1:nout){
      cat(sprintf("\n    t       x    u(x,t)
         u_ex(x,t)       u_err(x,t)\n"));
      for(ix in 1:nx){
        cat(sprintf("%5.1f%8.2f%10.5f%12.5f%13.6f\n",
           tout[it], xg[ix],
        u_plot[ix,it],ua_plot[ix,it],u_plot[ix,it]
           -ua_plot [ix,it]));
      }
    }
  }
```

Note again the use of two for's to step through t and x.

- The number of calls to fhn_1 is displayed at the end of the solution as a measure of the computational effort required to compute the solution.

```
#
# Calls to ODE routine
  cat(sprintf("\n\n ncall = %5d\n\n",ncall));
```

- The numerical solution of eq. (4.1a) is plotted against x with t as a parameter using matplot that produces solution curves as solid lines. The analytical solution is plotted as discrete points with matpoints

```
  #
  # Plot u numerical, analytical solution
    par(mfrow=c(1,1));
    matplot(x=xg,y=u_plot,type="l",xlab="x",ylab="u1
       (x,t),t=0,10,...,60",xlim=c(xl,xu),lty=1,
            main="u(x,t); solid - num, points - anal;
               t=0,10,...,60;",lwd=2);
    matpoints(x=xg,y=ua_plot,xlim=c(xl,xu),col="black",
       lwd=2)
```

par(mfrow=c(1,1)) specifies a 1×1 array of plots, that is, a single plot.

To complete the discussion of the programming, the IC function, u0_1, is in Listing 4.4.

```
  u0_1=function(t0){
#
# Function u0_1 sets the initial condition for the
# Fitzhugh-Nagumo equation
#
# IC from analytical solution
  uo=rep(0,nx);
  for(i in 1:nx){
    uo[i]=ua_1(xg[i],0);
  }
  return(c(uo));
  }
```

Listing 4.4 IC function u0_1 for eq. (4.1b).

Note the use of the analytical solution ua_1 from Listing 4.2a with $t = 0$. The IC vector is returned as uo.

This completes the programming of eqs. (4.1) and (4.2). We now consider the output from the main program of Listing 4.3.

4.4 Model Output

Abbreviated tabular numerical output for ncase=1 is given in Table 4.1.

TABLE 4.1 Abbreviated output for eqs. (4.1) and (4.2) from Listing 4.3, ncase=1.

```
a =  1.00   D =  1.00

> nrow(out)
[1] 7
> ncol(out)
[1] 102

  t        x     u(x,t)    u_ex(x,t)    u_err(x,t)
0.0   -60.00    1.00000      1.00000      0.000000
0.0   -59.20    1.00000      1.00000      0.000000
0.0   -58.40    1.00000      1.00000      0.000000
0.0   -57.60    1.00000      1.00000      0.000000
0.0   -56.80    1.00000      1.00000      0.000000
0.0   -56.00    1.00000      1.00000      0.000000
           .                                .
           .                                .
           .                                .
     Output for x = -55.20 to -12.80 removed
           .                                .
           .                                .
           .                                .
0.0   -12.00    0.99979      0.99979      0.000000
0.0   -11.20    0.99964      0.99964      0.000000
0.0   -10.40    0.99936      0.99936      0.000000
0.0    -9.60    0.99887      0.99887      0.000000
0.0    -8.80    0.99802      0.99802      0.000000
0.0    -8.00    0.99652      0.99652      0.000000
0.0    -7.20    0.99389      0.99389      0.000000
0.0    -6.40    0.98929      0.98929      0.000000
0.0    -5.60    0.98129      0.98129      0.000000
0.0    -4.80    0.96752      0.96752      0.000000
0.0    -4.00    0.94419      0.94419      0.000000
0.0    -3.20    0.90574      0.90574      0.000000
0.0    -2.40    0.84515      0.84515      0.000000
0.0    -1.60    0.75609      0.75609      0.000000
0.0    -0.80    0.63777      0.63777      0.000000
0.0     0.00    0.50000      0.50000      0.000000
```

(*continued*)

TABLE 4.1 (*Continued*)

```
  0.0    0.80   0.36223     0.36223     0.000000
  0.0    1.60   0.24391     0.24391     0.000000
  0.0    2.40   0.15485     0.15485     0.000000
  0.0    3.20   0.09426     0.09426     0.000000
  0.0    4.00   0.05581     0.05581     0.000000
          .                               .
          .                               .
          .                               .
       Output for x = 4.80 to 15.20 removed
          .                               .
          .                               .
          .                               .
  0.0   16.00   0.00001     0.00001     0.000000
  0.0   16.80   0.00001     0.00001     0.000000
  0.0   17.60   0.00000     0.00000     0.000000
  0.0   18.40   0.00000     0.00000     0.000000
  0.0   19.20   0.00000     0.00000     0.000000
  0.0   20.00   0.00000     0.00000     0.000000

    Output for t = 10, 20, 30, 40, 50 removed

    t       x    u(x,t)   u_ex(x,t)   u_err(x,t)
 60.0  -60.00   1.00000     1.00000     0.000004
 60.0  -59.20   0.99999     0.99999     0.000000
 60.0  -58.40   0.99999     0.99999     0.000001
 60.0  -57.60   0.99998     0.99998     0.000001
 60.0  -56.80   0.99996     0.99996     0.000002
 60.0  -56.00   0.99993     0.99993     0.000003
          .                               .
          .                               .
          .                               .
      Output for x = -55.20 to -48.40 removed
          .                               .
          .                               .
          .                               .
 60.0  -48.00   0.98109     0.98094     0.000143
 60.0  -47.20   0.96715     0.96693     0.000220
 60.0  -46.40   0.94360     0.94320     0.000403
 60.0  -45.60   0.90498     0.90414     0.000844
```

TABLE 4.1 (*Continued*)

```
60.0  -44.80  0.84443    0.84269    0.001742
60.0  -44.00  0.75572    0.75263    0.003089
60.0  -43.20  0.63769    0.63344    0.004250
60.0  -42.40  0.49960    0.49533    0.004266
60.0  -41.60  0.36119    0.35793    0.003263
60.0  -40.80  0.24282    0.24048    0.002340
60.0  -40.00  0.15416    0.15242    0.001734
60.0  -39.20  0.09391    0.09267    0.001236
60.0  -38.40  0.05566    0.05483    0.000826
60.0  -37.60  0.03241    0.03190    0.000509
60.0  -36.80  0.01867    0.01837    0.000297
60.0  -36.00  0.01068    0.01052    0.000166
          .                            .
          .                            .
          .                            .
     Output for x = -35.20 to 15.20 removed
          .                            .
          .                            .
          .                            .
60.0   16.00  0.00000    0.00000    0.000000
60.0   16.80 -0.00000    0.00000   -0.000000
60.0   17.60  0.00000    0.00000    0.000000
60.0   18.40  0.00000    0.00000    0.000000
60.0   19.20  0.00000    0.00000    0.000000
60.0   20.00  0.00000    0.00000    0.000001

ncall =   371
```

We can note the following details about this output.

- The dimensions of `out` are `out[7,102]` for seven output values of t, $t = 0, 10, \ldots, 60$, and $101 + 1 = 102$ as the second dimension to include t and the 101 ODEs.
- The output is for $t = 0, 60$. The output for the intermediate values of t ($t = 10, 20, 30, 40, 50$) is removed to conserve space.
- Within $t = 0, 60$ a portion of the output is removed to conserve space.

- The analytical and numerical solutions at $t = 0$ are the same as expected because both are based on eq. (4.1b). Also, the IC function of eq. (4.1b) has the value $u(x = 0, t = 0) = 1/(1 + \exp(0)) = 0.5$.
- The numerical solution of eqs. (4.1) and the analytical solution of eq. (4.2a) are in good agreement at $t = 60$. For example, from Table 4.1, at the point of maximum difference

```
t=60 x=-43.20,-42.60,-41.60

60.0   -43.20   0.63769     0.63344     0.004250
60.0   -42.40   0.49960     0.49533     0.004266
60.0   -41.60   0.36119     0.35793     0.003263
```

  This agreement between the two solutions is also reflected in Fig. 1.1.
- The traveling wave characteristic of eq. (4.2a) is reflected in the numerical solution. That is, the solution is a function of only the Lagrangian variable $x - vt$. We can explore this feature of the numerical solution numerically.

$$\frac{x}{\sqrt{2D}} + \left(a - \frac{1}{2}\right)t = \frac{1}{\sqrt{2D}}\left[x + \sqrt{2D}\left(a - \frac{1}{2}\right)t\right]$$

$$x - vt = x + \sqrt{2D}\left(a - \frac{1}{2}\right)t$$

or

$$v = -\sqrt{2D}\left(a - \frac{1}{2}\right)$$

For $a = D = 1$,

$$v = -\sqrt{2(1)}\left(1 - \frac{1}{2}\right) = -0.7071$$

Since v is negative, the traveling wave of eq. (4.2a) moves right to left (the direction of decreasing x) as reflected in Figs. 4.1. Generally, for $a < 1/2$, $v > 0$ and the front of eq. (4.2a) moves left to right, whereas for $a = 1/2$, $v = 0$ and the front does not

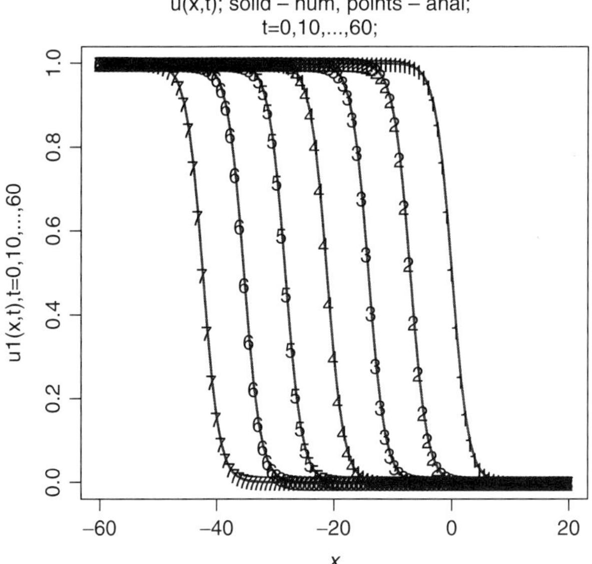

Figure 4.1 Figure 4.1 $u(x,t)$ versus x with t as a parameter, ncase=1.

move in t. The reader can easily verify these conclusions by changing the value of a in the main program of Listing 4.3.

- With the velocity $v = -0.7070$, the front will move a distance $(60)(0.7070) = 42.43$ with $t = 0$ to $t = 60$. This is confirmed approximately from Table 4.1 for $u(x = 0, t = 0)$ and $u(x = -42.40, t = 60)$.

```
  t=0

  0.0     0.00    0.50000      0.50000      0.000000

  t=60

 60.0   -42.40    0.49960      0.49533      0.004266
```

If the main program of Listing 4.3 is executed for the successive values of ncase=1,2,3,4,5, the following abbreviated output results.

```
ncase = 1, t=60 x=-43.20,-42.40,-41.60

60.0  -43.20    0.63769      0.63344      0.004250
60.0  -42.40    0.49960      0.49533      0.004266
```

```
60.0  -41.60   0.36119      0.35793      0.003263

ncase = 2, t=60 x=-43.20,-42.40,-41.60

60.0  -43.20   0.63769      0.63344      0.004250
60.0  -42.40   0.49960      0.49533      0.004266
60.0  -41.60   0.36119      0.35793      0.003263

ncase = 3, t=60 x=-43.20,-42.40,-41.60

60.0  -43.20   0.63769      0.63344      0.004250
60.0  -42.40   0.49960      0.49533      0.004266
60.0  -41.60   0.36119      0.35793      0.003263

ncase = 4, t=60 x=-43.20,-42.40,-41.60

60.0  -43.20   0.63769      0.63344      0.004250
60.0  -42.40   0.49960      0.49533      0.004266
60.0  -41.60   0.36119      0.35793      0.003263

ncase = 5, t=60 x=-43.20,-42.40,-41.60

60.0  -43.20   0.63769      0.63344      0.004250
60.0  -42.40   0.49960      0.49533      0.004266
60.0  -41.60   0.36119      0.35793      0.003263
```

The solution at the point of the maximum difference between the analytical and numerical solutions is invariant with the five alternative BCs programmed in `fhn_1` of Listing 4.1. This invariance results from a smooth solution, eq. (4.2a) with $D = 1$, that does not reach the boundaries (see Fig. 4.1).

To test this reasoning, the solution of eq. (4.1a) is repeated with a finite discontinuity IC rather than IC (4.1b).

4.5 Discontinuous Initial Condition

The revised main program for a unit step IC is in Listing 4.5.

```
#
# Access ODE integrator
```

```
  library("deSolve");
#
# Access functions for numerical solution
  setwd("c:/R/bme_pde/chap4");
  source("fhn_1.R");
  source("dss004.R");
#
# Level of output
#
#   ip = 1 - graphical (plotted) solutions
#            (u(x,t)) only
#
#   ip = 2 - numerical and graphical solutions
#
  ip=2;
#
# Alternative boundary conditions (BCs)
#
#   ncase = 1 - analytical Dirichlet BCs
#               (not used)
#
#   ncase = 2 - constant Dirichlet BCs
#
#   ncase = 3 - analytical Neumann BCs
#               (not used)
#
#   ncase = 4 - homogeneous Neumann BCs
#
#   ncase = 5 - no BCs
#
  ncase=2;
#
# Parameters
  a=1;D=1;
  cat(sprintf("\n\n a = %5.2f   D = %5.2f\n",a,D));
#
# Grid (in x)
  nx=101;xl=-60;xu=20;
  xg=seq(from=xl,to=xu,by=(xu-xl)/(nx-1));
#
# Independent variable for ODE integration
```

```
  nout=7;
  tout=seq(from=0,to=60,by=10);
#
# Initial condition (unit step)
  u0=rep(0,nx);t0=0;
  for(i in 1:101){
    if(i< 76){u0[i]=1;  }
    if(i==76){u0[i]=0.5;}
    if(i> 76){u0[i]=0;  }
  }
  ncall=0;
#
# ODE integration
  out=lsodes(y=u0,times=tout,func=fhn_1,parms=NULL)
  nrow(out)
  ncol(out)
#
# Arrays for plotting numerical solution
  u_plot=matrix(0,nrow=nx,ncol=nout);
 for(it in 1:nout){
   for(ix in 1:nx){
       u_plot[ix,it]=out[it,ix+1];
     }
  }
#
# Display numerical solution
  if(ip==2){
    for(it in 1:nout){
      cat(sprintf("\n    t        x    u(x,t)\n"));
      for(ix in 1:nx){
        cat(sprintf("%5.1f%8.2f%10.5f\n",tout[it],xg[ix],
           u_plot [ix,it]));
      }
    }
  }
#
# Calls to ODE routine
  cat(sprintf("\n\n ncall = %5d\n\n",ncall));
#
# Plot u numerical solution
  par(mfrow=c(1,1));
```

```
matplot(x=xg,y=u_plot,type="l",xlab="x",ylab="u1(x,t),
   t=0,10, ...,60",xlim=c(xl,xu),lty=1,main="u(x,t);
      t=0,10,...,60;",lwd=2);
```

Listing 4.5 Main program for eqs. (4.1) with unit step IC.

Listing 4.5 is similar to Listing 4.3, and the essential differences are discussed in the following.

- For a unit step IC (in place of eq. (4.2a)), an analytical solution is not available. Therefore, functions for only a numerical solution are accessed.

```
#
# Access functions for numerical solution
  setwd("c:/R/bme_pde/chap4");
  source("fhn_1.R");
  source("dss004.R");
```

- Also, `ncase=1,3` are not used in Listings 4.1 and 4.5 (an analytical solution is not available).

```
#
# Alternative boundary conditions (BCs)
#
#   ncase = 1 - analytical Dirichlet BCs
#               (not used)
#
#   ncase = 2 - constant Dirichlet BCs
#
#   ncase = 3 - analytical Neumann BCs
#               (not used)
#
#   ncase = 4 - homogeneous Neumann BCs
#
#   ncase = 5 - no BCs
#
  ncase=2;
```

- The parameters $a = 1, D = 1$, the interval in x, $-60 \leq x \leq 20$, and the interval in t, $0 \leq t \leq 60$ remain unchanged (from Listing 4.3).

- The unit step IC is at $x = 0$ (grid point 76).

```
#
# Initial condition (unit step)
  u0=rep(0,nx);t0=0;
  for(i in 1:101){
    if(i< 76){u0[i]=1;  }
    if(i==76){u0[i]=0.5;}
    if(i> 76){u0[i]=0;  }
  }
  ncall=0
```

- The ODE integration with `lsodes` is unchanged with the numerical solution placed in array `out`.
- Only the numerical solution in `out` is saved for plotting and then displayed for `ip=2` (because an analytical solution is not available).

```
#
# Arrays for plotting numerical solution
  u_plot=matrix(0,nrow=nx,ncol=nout);
 for(it in 1:nout){
   for(ix in 1:nx){
       u_plot[ix,it]=out[it,ix+1];
     }
  }
#
# Display numerical solution
  if(ip==2){
    for(it in 1:nout){
      cat(sprintf("\n    t        x    u(x,t)\n"));
      for(ix in 1:nx){
        cat(sprintf("%5.1f%8.2f%10.5f\n",tout[it],xg
           [ix],u_plot[ix,it]));
      }
    }
  }
```

- The number of calls to `fhn_1` is displayed as before (in Listing 4.3).

- A single plot of $u(x,t)$ against x with t as a parameter is produced with `matplot`.

```
#
# Plot u numerical solution
  par(mfrow=c(1,1));
  matplot(x=xg,y=u_plot,type="l",xlab="x",ylab="u1
     (x,t),t=0,10,...,60",xlim=c(xl,xu),lty=1,
        main="u(x,t);t=0,10,...,60;",lwd=2);
```

The numerical solution from Listing 4.5 is considered next. Abbreviated output for `ncase=2` is in Table 4.2.

We can note the following details about the output in Table 4.2.

- The unit step IC (at `t=0`) is confirmed.
- The solution is not a traveling wave in the sense that it is only a function of the Lagrangian variable $x - vt$ as in the case of eqs. (4.1b) and (4.2a). That is, the solution is not simply the IC displaced in x with increasing t.
- The computational effort is modest with `ncall` $= 422$, even with the discontinuous IC.

These properties are clearly displayed in Fig. 4.2. Also, this graphical output indicates that the discontinuous IC is accommodated without numerical distortion (e.g., oscillations), but rather, the solution is smooth. This is probably due in part to $D = 1$, a large enough value to smooth the solution.

For `ncase=4`, the abbreviated output is given in Table 4.3.

The solutions in Tables 4.2 and 4.3 are nearly identical, for example,

```
Table 4.2

60.0   -42.40   0.72149
60.0   -41.60   0.57801
60.0   -40.80   0.45277
```

TABLE 4.2 Abbreviated output for eq. (4.1a), unit step IC, ncase=2.

```
a =  1.00   D =  1.00

> nrow(out)
[1] 7
> ncol(out)
[1] 102

   t       x     u(x,t)
 0.0  -60.00    1.00000
 0.0  -59.20    1.00000
 0.0  -58.40    1.00000
 0.0  -57.60    1.00000
 0.0  -56.80    1.00000
 0.0  -56.00    1.00000
          .          .
          .          .
          .          .
 Output for x = -55.20
    to -4.80 removed
          .          .
          .          .
          .          .
 0.0    -4.00   1.00000
 0.0    -3.20   1.00000
 0.0    -2.40   1.00000
 0.0    -1.60   1.00000
 0.0    -0.80   1.00000
 0.0     0.00   0.50000
 0.0     0.80   0.00000
 0.0     1.60   0.00000
 0.0     2.40   0.00000
 0.0     3.20   0.00000
 0.0     4.00   0.00000
          .          .
          .          .
          .          .
```

TABLE 4.2 (*Continued*)

```
 Output for x = 4.80
   to 15.20 removed
      .         .
      .         .
      .         .
 0.0   16.00   0.00000
 0.0   16.80   0.00000
 0.0   17.60   0.00000
 0.0   18.40   0.00000
 0.0   19.20   0.00000
 0.0   20.00   0.00000

Output for t = 10, 20,
 30, 40, 50 removed

   t       x    u(x,t)
60.0  -60.00   1.00000
60.0  -59.20   0.99978
60.0  -58.40   0.99984
60.0  -57.60   0.99972
60.0  -56.80   1.00006
60.0  -56.00   0.99963
      .         .
      .         .
      .         .
 Output for x = -55.20
   to -48.80 removed
      .         .
      .         .
      .         .
60.0  -48.00   0.98984
60.0  -47.20   0.98957
60.0  -46.40   0.97284
60.0  -45.60   0.96389
60.0  -44.80   0.92545
60.0  -44.00   0.89092
60.0  -43.20   0.80658
60.0  -42.40   0.72149
60.0  -41.60   0.57801
```

(*continued*)

TABLE 4.2 (*Continued*)

```
 60.0  -40.80   0.45277
 60.0  -40.00   0.30635
 60.0  -39.20   0.21006
 60.0  -38.40   0.12448
 60.0  -37.60   0.07962
 60.0  -36.80   0.04356
 60.0  -36.00   0.02751
          .         .
          .         .
          .         .
  Output for x = -35.20
     to 15.20 removed
          .         .
          .         .
          .         .
 60.0   16.00  -0.00000
 60.0   16.80   0.00000
 60.0   17.60  -0.00000
 60.0   18.40  -0.00000
 60.0   19.20  -0.00000
 60.0   20.00   0.00000

 ncall =   422
```

```
 Table 4.3

 60.0  -42.40   0.72150
 60.0  -41.60   0.57800
 60.0  -40.80   0.45277
```

Therefore, the graphical solution for `ncase=4` is not included here. For `ncase=5`, the abbreviated output is given in Table 4.4.
We can note the following details about this output.

- The solution at the left end near $x = -60$ has a significant distortion (it does not remain close to 1 as with `ncase=2,4`).

```
 60.0  -60.00   1.16281
 60.0  -59.20   1.11858
 60.0  -58.40   1.08908
```

TABLE 4.3 Abbreviated output for eq. (4.1a), unit step IC, `ncase=4`.

```
a =  1.00   D =  1.00

> nrow(out)
[1] 7
> ncol(out)
[1] 102

Output for t = 0, 10, 20,
   30, 40, 50 removed

   t        x    u(x,t)
60.0  -60.00   1.00234
60.0  -59.20   0.99971
60.0  -58.40   1.00011
60.0  -57.60   0.99952
60.0  -56.80   1.00022
60.0  -56.00   0.99950
        .         .
        .         .
        .         .
 Output for x = -55.20
   to -48.80 removed
        .         .
        .         .
        .         .
60.0  -48.00   0.98982
60.0  -47.20   0.98959
60.0  -46.40   0.97282
60.0  -45.60   0.96390
60.0  -44.80   0.92544
60.0  -44.00   0.89093
60.0  -43.20   0.80657
60.0  -42.40   0.72150
60.0  -41.60   0.57800
60.0  -40.80   0.45277
60.0  -40.00   0.30635
60.0  -39.20   0.21006
60.0  -38.40   0.12448
```

(*continued*)

TABLE 4.3 (*Continued*)

```
 60.0  -37.60   0.07962
 60.0  -36.80   0.04356
 60.0  -36.00   0.02751
          .         .
          .         .
          .         .
  Output for x = -35.20
     to 15.20 removed
          .         .
          .         .
          .         .
 60.0   16.00  -0.00000
 60.0   16.80   0.00000
 60.0   17.60  -0.00000
 60.0   18.40   0.00000
 60.0   19.20  -0.00000
 60.0   20.00   0.00000

 ncall =   422
```

- In the interior, the solutions in Tables 4.3 and 4.4 differ by as much as in the third figure for some values of x, for example,

```
Table 4.3

60.0  -43.20   0.80657
60.0  -42.40   0.72150
60.0  -41.60   0.57800

Table 4.4

60.0  -43.20   0.80720
60.0  -42.40   0.72196
60.0  -41.60   0.57840
```

In summary, not using BCs for `ncase=5` in `fhn_1` of Listing 4.1 produces a substantial boundary effect (distortion) near $x = -60$.

TABLE 4.4 Abbreviated output for eq. (4.1a), unit step IC, `ncase=5`.

```
a =  1.00   D =  1.00

> nrow(out)
[1] 7
> ncol(out)
[1] 102

Output for t = 0, 10, 20,
   30, 40, 50 removed

   t        x     u(x,t)
60.0  -60.00   1.16281
60.0  -59.20   1.11858
60.0  -58.40   1.08908
60.0  -57.60   1.06796
60.0  -56.80   1.05291
60.0  -56.00   1.04088
        .         .
        .         .
        .         .
 Output for x = -55.20
   to -48.80 removed
        .         .
        .         .
        .         .
60.0  -48.00   0.99279
60.0  -47.20   0.99171
60.0  -46.40   0.97449
60.0  -45.60   0.96509
60.0  -44.80   0.92642
60.0  -44.00   0.89164
60.0  -43.20   0.80720
60.0  -42.40   0.72196
60.0  -41.60   0.57840
60.0  -40.80   0.45303
60.0  -40.00   0.30653
60.0  -39.20   0.21015
60.0  -38.40   0.12454
```

(continued)

TABLE 4.4 *(Continued)*

```
 60.0  -37.60   0.07965
 60.0  -36.80   0.04357
 60.0  -36.00   0.02752
          .         .
          .         .
          .         .
  Output for x = -35.20
     to 15.20 removed
          .         .
          .         .
          .         .
 60.0   16.00   0.00000
 60.0   16.80   0.00000
 60.0   17.60   0.00000
 60.0   18.40   0.00000
 60.0   19.20   0.00000
 60.0   20.00   0.00000

 ncall =   422
```

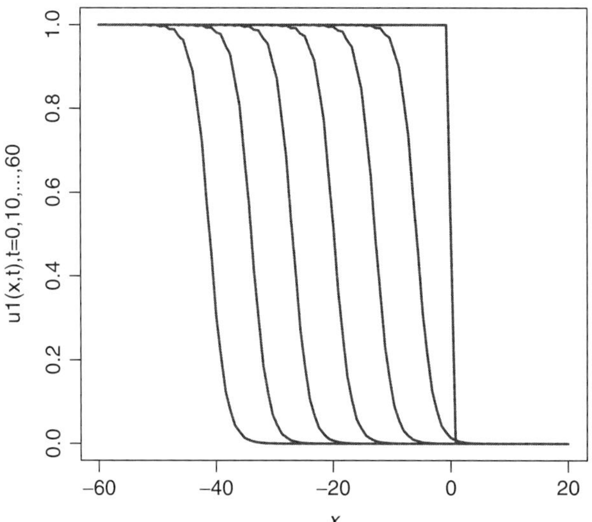

Figure 4.2 Figure 4.2 $u(x,t)$ versus x with t as a parameter, unit step IC, `ncase=2`.

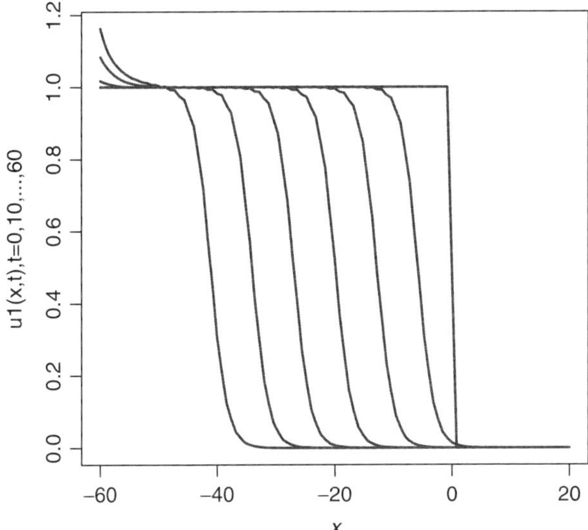

Figure 4.3 Figure 4.3 $u(x,t)$ versus x with t as a parameter, unit step IC, ncase=5.

In other words, this result indicates that BCs should be used. This boundary effect is evident in Fig. 4.3.

4.6 Conclusions

To conclude this study of the FHN equation, the cubic nonlinearity of eq. (4.1a) is easily included in the numerical solution of eq. (4.1a). In addition, the parameters a, D have a significant effect on the solution, for example, $a < 1/2, a > 1/2, a = 1/2$ for a traveling wave moving in the positive or negative x-direction with increasing t, or remaining invariant with t, respectively. Also, D smooths the solution and as it is decreased, numerical distortions might be expected, for example, unrealistic oscillations.

This conclusion suggests that the accuracy of the solutions should be investigated, for example, by changing the number of points in x (101 appears to be adequate for $a = 1, D = 1$) and the order of the numerical differentiation in x (dss004 appears to be adequate). These conclusions follow from the close agreement between the numerical and analytical solutions (as reflected in Fig. 4.1) and the smooth solutions from Listing 4.5 (as reflected in Fig. 4.2). However, more generally, some form of error analysis is essential when an analytical solution is not available (the usual case). The results of the application of h and p refinements (changes in the number of points in x and the spatial differentiator `dss004`) are not reported here to conserve space but can easily be carried out by the reader.

References

[1] Fitzhugh, R. (1955), Mathematical models of threshold phenomena in the nerve membrane, *Bull. Math. Biophysics*, **17**, 257-269.

[2] Griffiths, G.W., and W.E. Schiesser (2012), *Traveling Wave Analysis of Partial Differential Equations*, Elsevier, Burlington, MA.

[3] Hodgkin, A.L., and A.F. Huxley (1952), A quantitative description of membrane current and its application to conduction and excitation in nerve, *J. Physiol.*, **117**, 500-505.

[4] Murray, J.D. (2003), *Mathematical Biology, II: Spatial Models and Biomedical Applications*, 3rd Edition, Springer-Verlag, Berlin, Heidelberg.

[5] Nagumo, J., S. Arimoto, and S. Yoshizawa (1962), An active pulse transmission line simulating nerve axon, *Proc. IRE*, **50**, 2061-2070.

[6] Polyanin, A.D., and V.F. Zaitsev (2004), *Handbook of Nonlinear Partial Differential Equations*, Chapman & Hall/CRC, Boca Raton, FL.

CHAPTER 5

Anesthesia Spatiotemporal Distribution

5.1 Introduction

The PDE model discussed in this chapter pertains to spatial and temporal effects (distributions) of neuromuscular blocking agents used as anesthesia during surgery [1]. The variation of these rapid action drugs in space and time suggests a PDE model. Such a model was reported in [1] but with the limitation of a single linear PDE so that an analytical solution was possible. In the subsequent discussion, we consider the extension to a 2-PDE model that is not tractable by analytical methods so that a numerical solution is developed. The advantage of this approach is improved representation of the physiological system and response during the use of rapid action drugs.

The intent of this chapter is to demonstrate

- Formulation of a 2-PDE model that includes diffusion, convection, and binding of the drug.
- Specification of periodic boundary conditions and a delta (impulse, Dirac) function as an IC.
- Upwinding to accommodate the convection in a convection–diffusion PDE.
- Comparison of the computer implementation of the 2-PDE model with an earlier 1-PDE model.

Differential Equation Analysis in Biomedical Science and Engineering: Partial Differential Equation Applications with R, First Edition. William E. Schiesser.

- Effect of model structure and parameters on the spatiotemporal distribution of the drug;
- Extension of the model to include an inhomogeneous term in the PDE for the flowing drug concentration that generalizes the drug injection.

5.2 Two PDE Model

The following PDE model is based on a 1D circular domain with injection of the drug at one point along the domain and sampling of the plasma at another point to determine the time and spatial variation of the drug concentration [1]. The basic mass balances for the drug with fluid (plasma, flowing) concentration $u_1(x,t)$ and bound concentration $u_2(x,t)$ is a 2-PDE convection–diffusion system.

$$\frac{\partial u_1}{\partial t} = D_1 \frac{\partial^2 u_1}{\partial x^2} - \frac{\partial [v(x,t)u_1]}{\partial x} - g(t)u_1 - k_b u_1 (u_2^e - u_2) \quad (5.1a)$$

$$\frac{\partial u_2}{\partial t} = k_b u_1 (u_2^e - u_2) \quad (5.1b)$$

where

Mathematical term	Interpretation
u_1	flowing drug concentration
u_2	bound drug concentration
x	spatial coordinate in 1D circular domain
t	time
D_1	drug diffusivity
$v(x,t)$	fluid velocity
u_2^e	bound drug equilibrium (saturation) concentration
$g(t)$	function describing elimination rate
k_b	binding rate constant

The terms in eqs. (5.1) apply to a differential volume in x and are briefly described in the following.

- $\frac{\partial u_1}{\partial t}$: Rate of accumulation (positive derivative in t) or depletion (negative derivative in t) of the drug in the fluid.
- $D_1\frac{\partial^2 u_1}{\partial x^2}$: Net rate of drug diffusion into or out of the differential volume.
- $-\frac{\partial[v(x,t)u_1]}{\partial x}$: Net rate of drug convection into or out of the differential volume.
- $-g(t)u_1$: Rate of "elimination" of the drug (which originates in the 1-PDE model [1]). This effect, whatever may be its origin [1], is superseded in the 2-PDE model of eqs. (5.1) by the binding term (with k_b).
- $-k_b u_1(u_2^e - u_2)$: Rate of transfer of the drug from (or to) the fluid to (or from) the binding substrate. u_2^e is the saturation or limiting concentration of the drug on the substrate. The rate $u_1(u_2^e - u_2)$ is of a logistic form that approaches zero as $u_2 \rightarrow u_2^e$. The forward rate of binding is proportional to the product $u_1 u_2$, a nonlinear term that most likely precludes an analytical approach to the solution of eqs. (5.1). Also, the logistic form can provide binding (if $u_2 < u_2^e$) or debinding (if $u_2 > u_2^e$). At saturation, $u_2 = u_2^e$, no binding takes place.
- $\frac{\partial u_2}{\partial t}$: Rate of accumulation (binding, positive derivative in t) or depletion (unbinding, negative derivative in t) of the drug on the substrate.

Eq. (5.1a) is first order in t and second order in x. It, therefore, requires one initial condition (IC) and two boundary condition (BCs).

$$u_1(x, t = 0) = m_s\delta(x - x_i) \tag{5.2a}$$

$$u_1(x = 0, t) = u_1(x = L, t = 0) \tag{5.2b}$$

$$\frac{\partial u_1(x = L, t)}{\partial x} = \frac{\partial u_1(x = 0, t)}{\partial x} \tag{5.2c}$$

where

Mathematical term	Interpretation
x_i	point of drug injection
$\delta(x - x_i)$	delta function at x_i
m_s	magnitude (strength) of $\delta(x - x_i)$

The δ function of eq. (5.2a) is approximated numerically as a nonzero concentration (value of $u_1(x, t = 0)$) at one point corresponding to $x = x_i$. Everywhere else in x, this concentration is zero.

Eq. (5.2b) is a periodic BC [1] specifying that the concentration $u_1(x = 0, t)$ at $x = 0$ equals $u_1(x = L, t = 0)$ at the other end $x = L$ reflecting the circular geometry of the system, that is, for the circulation of the fluid in a closed system. Similarly, eq. (5.2c) specifies a periodic BC in the first derivative in x. We will observe that the use of periodic BCs is straightforward when considering the ODE/MOL routine.

Eq. (5.1b) is first order in t and therefore requires one IC.

$$u_2(x, t = 0) = 0 \tag{5.2d}$$

In other words, the substrate initially has no bound drug. Note also that for $k_b = 0$, eq. (5.1b) reduces to $\partial u_2/\partial t = 0$ indicating that the concentration $u_2(x, t)$ remains at zero. This follows since for this condition ($k_b = 0$), no transfer of the drug to the substrate takes place. This special case can serve as a check of the programming of eqs. (5.1).

5.2.1 Main Program

A main program for the MOL solution of eqs. (5.1) follows.

```
#
# Access ODE integrator
  library("deSolve");
```

```
#
# Access functions for analytical solutions
  setwd("c:/R/bme_pde/chap5");
  source("pharma_1.R");
  source("ge.R");
  source("vf.R");
  source("dss004.R");
  source("dss012.R");
  source("dss044.R");
#
# Level of output
#
#   ip = 1 - graphical (plotted) solutions
#            (u1(x,t), u2(x,t)) only
#
#   ip = 2 - numerical and graphical solutions
#
  ip=1;
#
# Grid in x
  nx=101;xl=0;xu=1;
  xg=seq(from=xl,to=xu,by=(xu-xl)/(nx-1));
#
# Grid in t
  nout=51;t0=0;tf=10;
  tout=seq(from=t0,to=tf,by=(tf-t0)/(nout-1));
#
# Parameters
  ncase=1;
  if(ncase==1){
    D1=3.0e-03;kb=1;u1e=1;ms=1;
  }
  if(ncase==2){
    D1=3.0e-03;kb=0;u1e=1;ms=1;
  }
#
# Display parameters
  cat(sprintf(
    "\n\n  D1 = %8.3e  kb = %6.3f  u1e = %6.3f
       ms = %6.3f\n",D1,kb,u1e,ms));
  Pe=vf(xg[51],0)*(xu-xl)/D1;
```

```
  cat(sprintf("\n Peclet number = %5.2f\n",Pe));
#
# IC
  u0=rep(0,2*nx);u10=rep(0,nx);u20=rep(0,nx);
  for(i in 1:nx){
    if(i==51){
      u10[i]=ms;
    }else{
      u10[i]=0;
    }
    u20[i]=0;
    u0[i]   =u10[i];
    u0[i+nx]=u20[i];
  }
  ncall=0;
#
# ODE integration
  out=lsodes(y=u0,times=tout,func=pharma_1,parms=NULL)
  nrow(out)
  ncol(out)
#
# Arrays for plotting numerical solution
  u1_xplot=matrix(0,nrow=nx,ncol=nout);
  u2_xplot=matrix(0,nrow=nx,ncol=nout);
  for(it in 1:nout){
    for(ix in 1:nx){
       u1_xplot[ix,it]=out[it,ix+1];
       u2_xplot[ix,it]=out[it,ix+1+nx];
    }
  }
#
# Display numerical solution (for t = 0, 2,...,10)
  if(ip==2){
    for(it in 1:nout){
      if((it-1)*(it-11)*(it-21)*(it-31)*(it-41)*
         (it-51)==0){
        cat(sprintf("\n\n     t       x   u1(x,t)
           u2(x,t)"));
        for(ix in 1:nx){
          cat(sprintf("\n%6.1f%7.3f%10.5f%10.5f",
              tout[it],xg[ix],u1_xplot[ix,it],u2_xplot
```

```
                  [ix,it]));
        }
      }
    }
  }
#
# Calls to ODE routine
  cat(sprintf("\n\n ncall = %5d\n\n",ncall));
#
# Plot u1, u2 numerical solutions
#
# vs x with t as a parameter, t = 0,0.2,...,10
  par(mfrow=c(1,1));
  matplot(x=xg,y=u1_xplot,type="l",xlab="x",
          ylab="u1(x,t), t=0,0.2,...,10",xlim=c(xl,xu),
             lty=1,main="u1(x,t); t=0,0.2,...,10;",lwd=2);
  par(mfrow=c(1,1));
  matplot(x=xg,y=u1_xplot[,-1],type="l",xlab="x",
          ylab="u1(x,t), t=0.2,0.4,...,10",xlim=c(xl,xu),
             lty=1,main="u1(x,t); t=0.2,0.4,...,10;",
                lwd=2);
  par(mfrow=c(1,1));
  matplot(x=xg,y=u2_xplot,type="l",xlab="x",
          ylab="u2(x,t), t=0,0.2,...,10",xlim=c(xl,xu),
             lty=1,main="u2(x,t); t=0,0.2,...,10;",lwd=2);
#
# vs t at x = 0.8, t = 0,0.2,...,10
  par(mfrow=c(1,1));
  u1_tplot=rep(0,nout);
  for(it in 1:nout){
    u1_tplot[it]=u1_xplot[81,it];
  }
  matplot(x=tout,y=u1_tplot,type="l",xlab="t",
          ylab="u1(x,t), x = 0.8",xlim=c(t0,tf),lty=1,
          main="u1(x,t); x = 0.8",lwd=2);
  par(mfrow=c(1,1));
  u2_tplot=rep(0,nout);
  for(it in 1:nout){
    u2_tplot[it]=u2_xplot[81,it];
  }
  matplot(x=tout,y=u2_tplot,type="l",xlab="x",
```

```
      ylab="u2(x,t), x = 0.8",xlim=c(t0,tf),lty=1,
      main="u2(x,t); x = 0.8",lwd=2);
```

Listing 5.1 Main program for eqs. (5.1).

We can observe the following details of Listing 5.1.

- The library of ODE integrators is accessed (`deSolve`).

```
#
# Access ODE integrator
  library("deSolve");
```

- Six routines are accessed for the MOL solution of eqs. (5.1).

```
#
# Access functions for analytical solutions
  setwd("c:/R/bme_pde/chap5");
  source("pharma_1.R");
  source("ge.R");
  source("vf.R");
  source("dss004.R");
  source("dss012.R");
  source("dss044.R");
```

  The programming and use of these routines is discussed subsequently.

- The level of output is specified with `ip`.

```
#
# Level of output
#
#   ip = 1 - graphical (plotted) solutions
#            (u1(x,t), u2(x,t)) only
#
#   ip = 2 - numerical and graphical solutions
#
  ip=2;
```

  For `ip=2`, the numerical output is for $t = 0, 2, \ldots, 10$.

- A grid of 101 points in x is specified over the interval $0 \le x \le 1$.

```
#
# Grid in x
  nx=101;xl=0;xu=1;
  xg=seq(from=xl,to=xu,by=(xu-xl)/(nx-1));
```

  This relatively large number of points in x was selected to achieve acceptable spatial resolution for the delta function IC of eq. (5.2a).

- A grid of 51 points in t is specified over the interval $0 \le t \le 10$.

```
#
# Grid in t
  nout=51;t0=0;tf=10;
  tout=seq(from=t0,to=tf,by=(tf-t0)/(nout-1));
```

  The relatively large number of points in t was selected to give smooth output as a function of t (at a particular value of x).

- Two cases are programmed (for ncase=1,2). For ncase=1, $k_b \neq 0$ in eqs. (5.1) so there is transfer of the drug to the substrate. For ncase=2, there is no transfer of the drug, and therefore, from eq. (5.1b), $u_2(x,t)$ remains at its IC (eq. (5.2d)); this serves as a test of the coding of eqs. (5.1).

```
#
# Parameters
  ncase=1;
  if(ncase==1){
    D1=3.0e-03;kb=1;u1e=1;ms=1;
  }
  if(ncase==2){
    D1=3.0e-03;kb=0;u1e=1;ms=1;
  }
```

  The choice of the numerical values of the parameters is explained later (in combination with the velocity $v(x,t)$ in eq. (5.1a) set in function vf discussed subsequently).

- The parameters are displayed. Also, the Peclet number, `Pe`, is computed and displayed (using the velocity function `vf`).

```
#
# Display parameters
  cat(sprintf(
    "\n\n  D1 = %8.3e  kb = %6.3f  u1e = %6.3f
       ms = %6.3f\n",D1,kb,u1e,ms));
  Pe=vf(xg[51],0)*(xu-xl)/D1;
  cat(sprintf("\n Peclet number = %5.2f\n",Pe));
```

  Briefly, `Pe` can be considered as the ratio of convective transport from the numerator `vf(xg[26],0)*(xu-xl)` to diffusive transport from the denominator `D1`. This ratio is approximately `Pe` = 25 corresponding to the values in [1] as explained later. With the present programming in `vf` (discussed subsequently), the velocity $v(x,t)$ in eq. (5.1a) is constant (and the midpoint in x is used, i.e., `xg[51]` with $t = 0$ in the call to `vf`). However, the velocity can be programmed as a function of x and t in `vf` if this is considered an important effect.

- ICs (5.2a) and (5.2d) are programmed. Note in particular the approximation of the delta function in eq. (5.2a) at $x = x_i = 0.5$ (`i=51`).

```
#
# IC
  u0=rep(0,2*nx);u10=rep(0,nx);u20=rep(0,nx);
  for(i in 1:nx){
    if(i==51){
      u10[i]=ms;
    }else{
      u10[i]=0;
    }
    u20[i]=0;
    u0[i]   =u10[i];
    u0[i+nx]=u20[i];
  }
  ncall=0;
```

The initial values of u_1, u_2 are then placed in a single vector, u0, for use as an input to the ODE integrator, lsodes. The length of this IC vector informs lsodes how many ODEs are to be integrated ((2)(101) = 202). Finally, the number of calls to the ODE routine pharma_1 (considered later) is initialized.

- The ODEs are integrated by a call to lsodes. The dimensions of the solution array out are displayed as a check (discussed with the output later).

```
#
# ODE integration
  out=lsodes(y=u0,times=tout,func=pharma_1,
     parms=NULL)
  nrow(out)
  ncol(out)
```

Note the use of the IC array, u0, the vector of output values of t, tout, and the ODE function, pharma_1. y,times,func,parms are reserved names (parms is unused).

- The numerical solution in the 2D array out is placed in two 2D arrays, u1_xplot[ix,it] and u2_xplot[ix,it], for plotting as a function of x.

```
#
# Arrays for plotting numerical solution
  u1_xplot=matrix(0,nrow=nx,ncol=nout);
  u2_xplot=matrix(0,nrow=nx,ncol=nout);
  for(it in 1:nout){
    for(ix in 1:nx){
       u1_xplot[ix,it]=out[it,ix+1];
       u2_xplot[ix,it]=out[it,ix+1+nx];
    }
  }
```

Note the offset 1 for the second subscript of out, e.g., ix+1. This is required because the first value of this subscript is used for t, that is, out[it,1] contains t so the first ODE dependent variable is in out[it,2] (this is an operational property of lsodes).

- For ip=2, the numerical solution is displayed at $t = 0, 2, \ldots, 10$ (by using the index it in the if). This was done because the numerical solution in out is for 51 values of t that displays excessive numerical output but is required for graphical (plotted) output.

```
#
# Display numerical solution (for t = 0, 2,...,10)
  if(ip==2){
    for(it in 1:nout){
      if((it-1)*(it-11)*(it-21)*(it-31)*(it-41)*
         (it-51)==0){
        cat(sprintf("\n\n     t       x   u1(x,t)
           u2(x,t)"));
        for(ix in 1:nx){
          cat(sprintf("\n%6.1f%7.3f%10.5f%10.5f",
              tout[it],xg[ix],u1_xplot[ix,it],
                 u2_xplot[ix,it]));
        }
      }
    }
  }
```

- The number of calls to pharma_1 at the end of the solution is displayed as an indication of the computational effort required to compute the solution.

```
#
# Calls to ODE routine
  cat(sprintf("\n\n ncall = %5d\n\n",ncall));
```

- The plotting is in two forms, (i) parametric plots in t and (ii) plots at a particular x. For the first, the coding for three plots using matplot is

```
#
# Plot u1, u2 numerical solutions
#
# vs x with t as a parameter, t = 0,0.2,...,10
  par(mfrow=c(1,1));
```

```
  matplot(x=xg,y=u1_xplot,type="l",xlab="x",
          ylab="u1(x,t), t=0,0.2,...,10",xlim=c
             (xl,xu),lty=1,main="u1(x,t);
                t=0,0.2,...,10;",lwd=2);
  par(mfrow=c(1,1));
  matplot(x=xg,y=u1_xplot[,-1],type="l",xlab="x",
          ylab="u1(x,t), t=0.2,0.4,...,10",xlim=c
             (xl,xu),lty=1,main="u1(x,t);
                t=0.2,0.4,...,10;",lwd=2);
  par(mfrow=c(1,1));
  matplot(x=xg,y=u2_xplot,type="l",xlab="x",
          ylab="u2(x,t), t=0,0.2,...,10",xlim=c
             (xl,xu),lty=1,main="u2(x,t);
                t=0,0.2,...,10;",lwd=2);
```

`par(mfrow=c(1,1))` specifies a 1×1 array of plots, that is, single plots. The arguments for `matplot` are largely self-explanatory (note in particular the `x,y` or horizontal–vertical variables). The second plot is an attempt to obtain better resolution by avoiding the approximate delta function at $t = 0$ (IC (5.2a)). This is accomplished by plotting `y=u1_xplot[,-1]`, that is, by not using the first value of the second subscript (in t). The resulting plots are in Figs. 5.1–5.3.

- Two plots are produced for $u_1(x = 0.8, t)$, $u_2(x = 0.8, t)$ corresponding to point `81` in x ($(81 - 1)/(101 - 1) = 0.8$).

```
#
# vs t at x = 0.8, t = 0,0.2,...,10
  par(mfrow=c(1,1));
  u1_tplot=rep(0,nout);
  for(it in 1:nout){
    u1_tplot[it]=u1_xplot[81,it];
  }
  matplot(x=tout,y=u1_tplot,type="l",xlab="t",
          ylab="u1(x,t), x = 0.8",xlim=c(t0,tf),
             lty=1,main="u1(x,t); x = 0.8",lwd=2);
  par(mfrow=c(1,1));
  u2_tplot=rep(0,nout);
  for(it in 1:nout){
```

```
    u2_tplot[it]=u2_xplot[81,it];
  }
  matplot(x=tout,y=u2_tplot,type="l",xlab="x",
          ylab="u2(x,t), x = 0.8",xlim=c(t0,tf),
             lty=1,main="u2(x,t); x = 0.8",lwd=2);
```

Recall that the drug injection is at $x = 0.5$ or point 51 (from the previous programming of IC (5.2a)), so the response at $x = 0.8$ reflects the convection and diffusion of the drug in moving from $x = 0.5$ to $x = 0.8$. The response at other values of x can easily be selected. The graphical output from these $u_1(x = 0.8, t), u_2(x = 0.8, t)$ plots is in Figs. 5.4 and 5.5.

The additional routines are considered next, starting with the ODE routine, `pharma_1`, called by `lsodes`.

5.2.2 ODE Routine

The MOL/ODE routine for eqs. (5.1) is in Listing 5.2.

```
  pharma_1=function(t,u,parms){
#
# Function pharma_1 computes the t derivative vector
# of the u1,u2 vectors
#
# One vector to two vectors
  u1=rep(0,nx);u2=rep(0,nx);
  for(i in 1:nx){
    u1[i]=u[i];
    u2[i]=u[i+nx];
  }
#
# Boundary conditions
  u1[1]=u1[nx];
  u1x=dss004(xl,xu,nx,u1);
  u1x[nx]=u1x[1];
  nl=1;nu=2;
#
# u1xx
  u1xx=dss044(xl,xu,nx,u1,u1x,nl,nu);
```

```
#
# (v*u1)x
  vu1=rep(0,nx);
  for(i in 1:nx){
    vu1[i]=vf(xg[i],t)*u1[i];
  }
# vu1x=dss004(xl,xu,nx,vu1);
  vu1x=dss012(xl,xu,nx,vu1,1);
#
# PDEs
  u1t=rep(0,nx);u2t=rep(0,nx);
  for(i in 1:nx){
    u1t[i]=D1*u1xx[i]-vu1x[i]-ge(t)*u1[i]-kb*u1[i]*
       (u1e-u1[i]);
    u2t[i]=kb*u1[i]*(u1e-u1[i]);
  }
  u1t[1]=0;
#
# Two vectors to one vector
  ut=rep(0,2*nx);
  for(i in 1:nx){
    ut[i]   =u1t[i];
    ut[i+nx]=u2t[i];
  }
#
# Increment calls to pharma_1
  ncall <<- ncall+1;
#
# Return derivative vector
  return(list(c(ut)));
}
```

Listing 5.2 ODE routine pharma_1 for eqs. (5.1).

We can note the following details about pharma_1.

- The function is defined. The second input argument u is a vector of 202 dependent variables that is sized by the IC array u0 defined in the main program of Listing 5.1.

```
pharma_1=function(t,u,parms){
```

```
#
# Function pharma_1 computes the t derivative vector
# of the u1,u2 vectors
```

- u is placed in two vectors of length 101 to facilitate the programming of eqs. (5.1).

```
#
# One vector to two vectors
  u1=rep(0,nx);u2=rep(0,nx);
  for(i in 1:nx){
    u1[i]=u[i];
    u2[i]=u[i+nx];
  }
```

- The periodic BCs of eqs. (5.2b) and (5.2c) are programmed. dss004 is used to calculate the derivative $\partial u_1/\partial x$ so that BC (5.2c) can be applied.

```
#
# Boundary conditions
  u1[1]=u1[nx];
  u1x=dss004(xl,xu,nx,u1);
  u1x[nx]=u1x[1];
  nl=1;nu=2;
```

  BC (5.2b) at $x = 0$ specifies $u_1(x = 0, t)$ (u1[1]) so that it is Dirichlet (nl=1). BC (5.2c) at $x = L$ specifies $\partial u_1(x = L, t)/\partial x$ (u1x[nx]) and is therefore Neumann (nu=2).
- The diffusion derivative in eq. (5.1a), $\partial^2 u_1)/\partial x^2$ (u1xx), is computed by dss044. That is, u1xx is a 101-vector.

```
#
# u1xx
  u1xx=dss044(xl,xu,nx,u1,u1x,nl,nu);
```

  Note that the BC derivative u1x[nx] is an input to dss044.
- The convection derivative $\partial[v(x, t)u_1]/\partial x$ in eq. (5.1a) (vu1x) is computed by dss012.

```
#
# (v*u1)x
  vu1=rep(0,nx);
  for(i in 1:nx){
    vu1[i]=vf(xg[i],t)*u1[i];
  }
# vu1x=dss004(xl,xu,nx,vu1);
  vu1x=dss012(xl,xu,nx,vu1,1);
```

First, the product $v(x,t)u_1$ is computed in a `for`, which illustrates the ease of including a variable coefficient ($v(x,t)$) in the analysis (function `vf` is discussed next). Note in particular how x and t can vary in $v(x,t)$ (although for the present case, v is a constant).

Since eq. (5.1a) is strongly convective (this will be confirmed when the output is discussed), a centered FD approximation such as in `dss004` cannot be used ([3], Chap 1). Rather, some upwinding is required. `dss012` is a library differentiator with two-point upwind finite differences that ensure that the numerical solution does not oscillate unrealistically (this would occur with centered FDs as in `dss004` for PDEs with substantial convection). Note that a fifth argument is used in `dss012` to specify the direction of the flow, in this case, in the positive x-direction; only the sign (and not the value) of this fifth argument is used to specify the direction of the flow (the direction of the upwinding).

- Eqs. (5.1) are programmed in a `for` with index `i` for $0 \leq x \leq 1$.

```
#
# PDEs
  u1t=rep(0,nx);u2t=rep(0,nx);
  for(i in 1:nx){
    u1t[i]=D1*u1xx[i]-vu1x[i]-ge(t)*u1[i]-kb*u1[i]*
        (u1e-u1[i]);
    u2t[i]=kb*u1[i]*(u1e-u1[i]);
  }
  u1t[1]=0;
```

The correspondence of this programming with eqs. (5.1) is clear, which is an advantage of the numerical approach. The result is $\partial u_1/\partial t, \partial u_2/\partial t$ in arrays `u1t,u2t`. Note the use of the function

ge for the variable coefficient of the elimination term $-g(t)u_1$ in eq. (5.1a). Also, the binding of the drug takes place at the rate kb*u1[i]*(u1e-u1[i]) as stated in eqs. (5.1).
Since the BC at $x = 0$ is Dirichlet ($u_1(x = 0, t)$ is coded as u1[1]=u1[nx]), u1t[1]=0 is used to prevent the ODE integrator from moving $u_1(x = 0, t)$ away from the BC value. In other words, u1t[1]=0 serves as the ODE for u_1 at $x = 0$. At $x = L$, the BC is Neumann and therefore the PDE for $u_1(x = L, t)$, eq. (5.1a), is used to define an ODE at $x = L$; that is, the derivative u1t[nx] is computed from the PDE, eq. (5.1a), at $x = L$.

- The two derivative vectors are placed in a single vector ut of length 2*nx $=$ 202 for return to lsodes.

```
#
# Two vectors to one vector
  ut=rep(0,2*nx);
  for(i in 1:nx){
    ut[i]   =u1t[i];
    ut[i+nx]=u2t[i];
  }
```

- The counter for the calls to pharma_1 is incremented and returned to the main program of Listing 5.1 with <<- (ncall is a local variable not available to the main program without using <<-).

```
#
# Increment calls to pharma_1
  ncall <<- ncall+1;
```

- The derivative vector ut is returned to lsodes as a list (as required by lsodes).

```
#
# Return derivative vector
  return(list(c(ut)));
}
```

The final } concludes pharma_1.

The functions vf and ge used in the preceding programming of eqs. (5.1) are considered next.

5.2.3 Other PDE Routines

Function vf is in Listing 5.3.

```
  vf=function(x,t){
#
# Function vf computes the fluid (blood plasma) velocity
# as a function of x and t
#
  v=0.075;
  return(c(v));
  }
```

Listing 5.3 PDE routine vf.

In this case, the velocity in eq. (5.1a) is set to the constant value 0.075, but v could be programmed as a function of x and t. Note that the velocity is returned as a numerical vector with one element.

The value v=0.075 was selected so that the Peclet number is

$$Pe = \frac{v(x,t)L}{D_1} = \frac{(0.075)(1)}{0.003} = 25$$

$L = 1$ and $D_1 = 0.003$ are the values used in Listing 5.1. $Pe = 25$ corresponds approximately to the values reported by Lafrance et al. [1] ($\nu = 24.185, 21.770$ in Table 1). This value for Pe means that the PDE system of eqs. (5.1) is substantially convective (relative to diffusive) and thus the upwinding in dss012 is used in pharma_1. The Peclet number from [1] was devised in the following way (using the notation in [1]).

$$L = (v)(t_1 - t_0);\ D = \frac{(v^2)(t_1 - t_0)}{\nu}$$

Thus,

$$Pe = \frac{L v}{D} = \frac{(v)(t_1 - t_0)(v)}{(v^2)(t_1 - t_0)/\nu} = \nu$$

In other words, ν in [1] is Pe.

Function ge is in Listing 5.4.

```
  ge=function(t){
```

```
#
# Function ge computes the variable coefficient for the
# elimination function
#
  if(ncase==1){
    g=0;
  }
  if(ncase==2){
    rho=1.215;P=4246.230;Q=1010.330;sig=0.084;
    exp1=exp(-rho*t);
    exp2=exp(-sig*t);
    g=(rho*P*exp1+sig*Q*exp2)/(P*exp1+Q*exp2);
  }
  return(c(g));
  }
```

Listing 5.4 Routine ge used in Listing 5.2 (for $g(t)$ of eq. (5.1a)).

The two cases, ncase=1,2, used in the main program of Listing 5.1 are programmed. For ncase=1, the elimination function in eq. (5.1a) is not used (g=0) so that only the drug binding rate with k_r is used in the calculations. For ncase=2, the variable coefficient reported in [1] is used.

$$g(t) = \frac{\rho P e^{-\rho t} + \sigma Q e^{-\sigma t}}{P e^{-\rho t} + Q e^{-\sigma t}}$$

with values of ρ, P, Q, σ selected from [1]. Since the $g(t)$ function is relatively difficult to visualize numerically, the following small program computes and tabulates numerical values of $g(t)$.

```
setwd("c:/R/bme_pde/chap5")
source("ge.R")
tout=seq(from=0,to=20,by=2);
nout=11;gt=rep(0,nout);ncase=2;
for(it in 1:nout){
  gt[it]=ge(tout[it]);
  cat(sprintf("\n t = %5.1f  g(t) = %8.5f",tout[it],
     gt[it]));
}
```

Listing 5.5 Main program to evaluate ge of Listing 5.4.

TABLE 5.1 Output from Listing 5.5.

```
t =   0.0  g(t) =  0.998
t =   1.0  g(t) =  0.735
t =   2.0  g(t) =  0.428
t =   3.0  g(t) =  0.224
t =   4.0  g(t) =  0.133
t =   5.0  g(t) =  0.100
t =   6.0  g(t) =  0.089
t =   7.0  g(t) =  0.086
t =   8.0  g(t) =  0.085
t =   9.0  g(t) =  0.084
t =  10.0  g(t) =  0.084
```

This main program is largely self-explanatory. Note the use of the function `ge` accessed with the `source` statement. Also, `ncase=2` for use in function `ge`. The output from Listing 5.5 is in Table 5.1.

This output indicates that for $0 \leq t \leq 10$ and the numerical values of the parameters in Listing 5.4, $g(t)$ in eq. (5.1a) is bounded approximately as $0.084 \leq g(t) \leq 1$ (which gives an indication of the effect of $g(t)$ in eq. (5.1a)).

5.2.4 Model Output

The output from the preceding routines in Listings 5.1–5.4 is now reviewed. The abbreviated numerical output is given in Table 5.2 for `ncase=1`.

We can note the following details about this numerical output.

- $k_b = 1$ corresponding to `ncase=1` so that drug transfer to the substrate takes place.
- $Pe = 25$ as discussed previously so that eq. (5.1a) has a substantial convective component in the term $\partial[v(x,t)u_1]/\partial x$.
- Array `out` in Listing 5.1 has a column dimension of `203` as expected, that is, `2*101+1=203` to include the value of t.

TABLE 5.2 Abbreviated output from Listing 5.1 for ncase=1.

```
D1 = 3.000e-03  kb =  1.000  u1e =  1.000
   ms =  1.000

Peclet number = 25.00

> nrow(out)
[1] 51
> ncol(out)
[1] 203

    t      x    u1(x,t)   u2(x,t)
  0.0  0.000   0.00000   0.00000
  0.0  0.010   0.00000   0.00000
  0.0  0.020   0.00000   0.00000
  0.0  0.030   0.00000   0.00000
  0.0  0.040   0.00000   0.00000
  0.0  0.050   0.00000   0.00000
         .                  .
         .                  .
         .                  .
  Output for x = 0.060 to 0.440
             removed
         .                  .
         .                  .
         .                  .
  0.0  0.450   0.00000   0.00000
  0.0  0.460   0.00000   0.00000
  0.0  0.470   0.00000   0.00000
  0.0  0.480   0.00000   0.00000
  0.0  0.490   0.00000   0.00000
  0.0  0.500   1.00000   0.00000
  0.0  0.510   0.00000   0.00000
  0.0  0.520   0.00000   0.00000
  0.0  0.530   0.00000   0.00000
  0.0  0.540   0.00000   0.00000
  0.0  0.550   0.00000   0.00000
```

TABLE 5.2 (*Continued*)

```
        .                 .
        .                 .
        .                 .
 Output for x = 0.560 to 0.940
             removed
        .                 .
        .                 .
        .                 .
 0.0  0.950   0.00000   0.00000
 0.0  0.960   0.00000   0.00000
 0.0  0.970   0.00000   0.00000
 0.0  0.980   0.00000   0.00000
 0.0  0.990   0.00000   0.00000
 0.0  1.000   0.00000   0.00000
        .                 .
        .                 .
        .                 .
 Output for t = 2 to 8 removed
        .                 .
        .                 .
        .                 .
   t      x   u1(x,t)   u2(x,t)
10.0  0.000   0.00000   0.00091
10.0  0.010   0.00000   0.00083
10.0  0.020   0.00000   0.00076
10.0  0.030   0.00000   0.00069
10.0  0.040   0.00000   0.00063
10.0  0.050   0.00000   0.00057
        .                 .
        .                 .
        .                 .
 Output for x = 0.060 to 0.940
             removed
        .                 .
        .                 .
        .                 .
10.0  0.950   0.00000   0.00117
```

(*continued*)

TABLE 5.2 *(Continued)*

```
10.0  0.960   0.00000   0.00108
10.0  0.970   0.00000   0.00101
10.0  0.980   0.00000   0.00096
10.0  0.990   0.00000   0.00093
10.0  1.000   0.00000   0.00091

ncall =   394
```

- IC (5.2a) is confirmed in the output at $x = 0.5, t = 0$, that is, the delta function of eq. (5.2a) is represented by the following output.

```
  t       x    u1(x,t)   u2(x,t)
0.0   0.500   1.00000   0.00000
```

  Note that this single `1.00000` in all of the `2*101=202` IC values is what drives the entire model away from zero! In a physical sense, we would expect this `1.00000` to be "diluted" to lower values with convection, diffusion, and binding, and this is what happens as observed in the output of Table 5.2 for $t = 10$. Note in particular that the drug transfer to the substrate, that is, the zero values of $u_2(x, t = 0)$ change to the nonzero values of $u_2(x, t = 10)$. A clearer picture of this dispersion of the drug is presented in the following graphical output (Figs. 5.1–5.5).
- The computational effort is modest with `ncall = 394`.

The graphical output from Listing 5.1 is in Figs. 5.1–5.5. These figures are briefly discussed next. The approximation of the delta function in BC (5.2b) is clear. Note that the maximum value of 1 decreases rapidly (for $t > 0$) to smaller values because of convection, diffusion, and binding. The density of the plots is due to `nout=51` values of t, $t = 0, 0.2, \ldots, 10$. This large number of t values was used to give acceptable resolution in Figs. 5.4 and 5.5. The successive curves appear to reach a steady-state (time invariant) solution. Since the delta function (at $t = 0$) dominates Fig. 5.1, the solution for

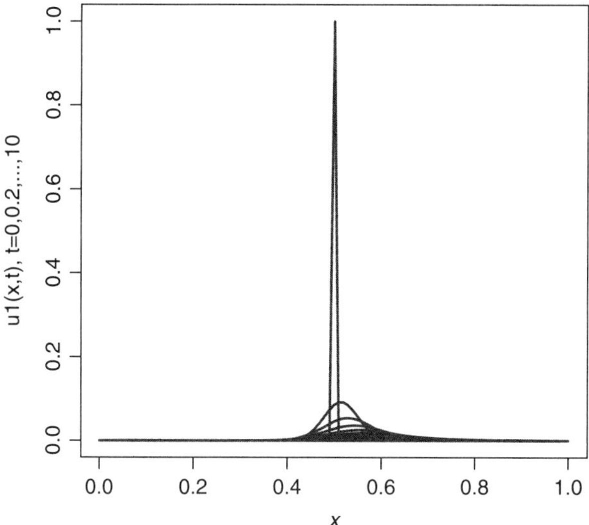

Figure 5.1 $u_1(x,t)$ versus x with t as a parameter, $t = 0, 0.2, \ldots, 10$, ncase=1.

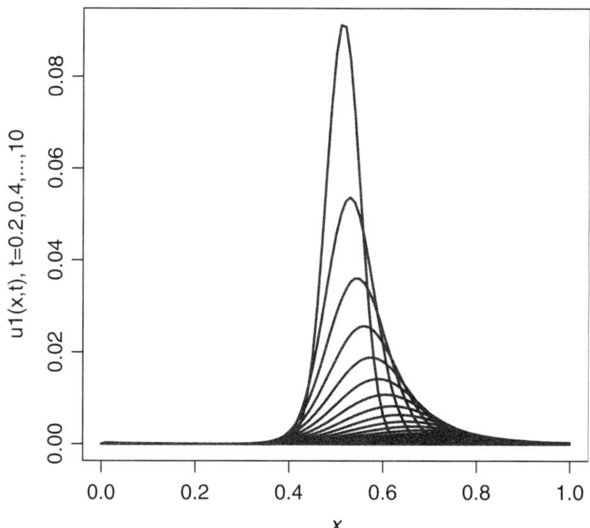

Figure 5.2 $u_1(x,t)$ versus x with t as a parameter, $t = 0.2, 0.4, \ldots, 10$, ncase=1.

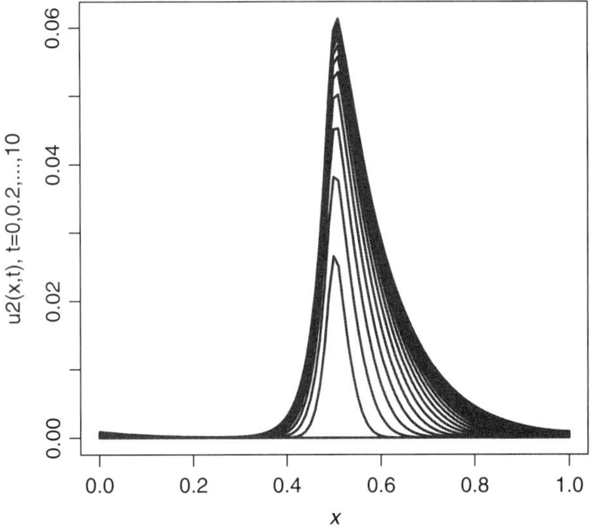

Figure 5.3 $u_2(x,t)$ versus x with t as a parameter, $t = 0, 0.2, \ldots, 10$, ncase=1.

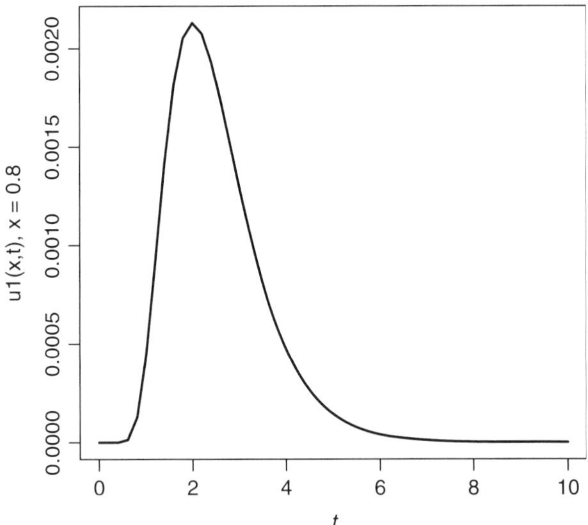

Figure 5.4 $u_1(x,t)$ versus t at $x = 0.8$, ncase=1.

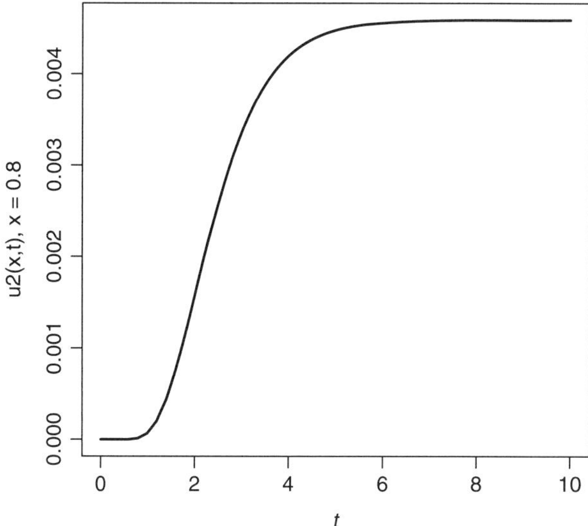

Figure 5.5 $u_2(x,t)$ versus t at $x = 0.8$, ncase=1.

$u_1(x,t)$ is replotted in Fig. 5.2 without $t = 0$ $(t = 0.2, 0.4, \ldots, 10)$. The reduction in the successive peaks with increasing t is clear. The uptake (binding) of the drug on the substrate, starting with a zero value $(u_2(x,t=0) = 0)$ is clear. The peaks increase from bottom to top and appear to reach a steady state (at $t = 10$). The solution in Fig. 5.4 for $x = 0.8$ corresponds to $0.8 - 0.5 = 0.3$ units in x away from the point of drug injection. $x = 0.8$ is suggested (estimated) from the figures in [1] for the point of fluid (blood plasma) sampling. The substrate concentration $u_2(x = 0.8, t)$ in Fig. 5.5 appears to reach a steady-state level.

To conclude this discussion of the output, Fig. 5.4 is repeated with ncase=2 in Listing 5.1 (corresponding to no substrate binding so $u_2(x,t)$ remains at the initial value of t). The solution in Fig. 5.4, $u_1(x = 0.8, t)$, has a maximum value of approximately 0.0022 with a relatively fast response in t, where as in Fig. 5.6, the maximum value of $u_1(x = 0.8, t)$ is approximately 0.0042 with a relatively slow response in t. These differences can be attributed to the difference in the 2-PDE (ncase=1) and 1-PDE (ncase=2) models. The 2-PDE model is considered physically to be a better representation of the

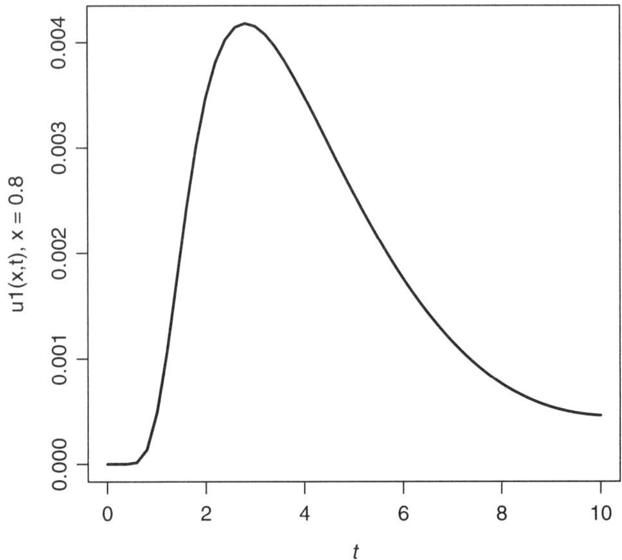

Figure 5.6 $u_1(x,t)$ versus t at $x = 0.8$, ncase=2.

fluid spatiotemporal dynamics because of the binding of the drug. In particular, the faster response in Fig. 5.4 can be attributed to the binding of the drug.

5.3 Conclusions

The addition of binding to the 1-PDE model of Lafrance et al. [1] was straightforward. However, the addition of a second PDE, and the use of the nonlinear logistic binding rate, precludes an analytical solution to eqs. (5.1).

Also, as a word of caution, Fig. 5.1 indicates the very sharp variation in the solution for small t. In fact, if the calculation of the derivative $\partial^2 u_1(x,t=0)/\partial x^2$ in eq. (5.1a) is considered, it would seem that a numerical solution would not be possible (the second derivative of the delta function is required at $t = 0$). This is in contrast with the analytical approach for which the delta function actually makes the derivation of analytical solutions easier, for example, the evaluation of integrals is simplified. Although a numerical solution could be computed, as reflected in Table 5.2, the computations may be very sensitive to changes in the model parameters, including the strength of the delta function, `ms`. Thus, experimentation with the model might produce a situation for which a numerical solution cannot be computed (again, it seems rather remarkable that any numerical solutions could be computed with the approximation of the delta function programmed as the IC in Listing 5.1, especially when considering the hyperbolic–parabolic, or convective–diffusive, character of eq. (5.1a)).

Finally, a discussion of the numerical approximation of the delta function in PDE solutions is given in [2], Chapter 3. This discussion includes the selection of the strength of the delta function, for example, `ms`, so that analytical and numerical solutions agree.

5.4 Model Extension

The preceding model of eqs. (5.1) and (5.2) includes delta function IC (5.2a) for the drug injection. While a delta function is convenient for an analytical analysis, it is relatively difficult to represent numerically, and physically may not be realistic. We therefore consider an extension of the preceding model of eqs. (5.1) and (5.2), which has an inhomogeneous term added to eq. (5.1a) to reflect the drug injection that can have a general form in x and t. The model then becomes

$$\frac{\partial u_1}{\partial t} = D_1 \frac{\partial^2 u_1}{\partial x^2} - \frac{\partial [v(x,t)u_1]}{\partial x} - k_b u_1 (u_2^e - u_2) + g_s(x,t) \tag{5.3a}$$

$$\frac{\partial u_2}{\partial t} = k_b u_1 (u_2^e - u_2) \tag{5.3b}$$

$$u_1(x, t = 0) = 0 \tag{5.4a}$$

$$u_1(x = 0, t) = u_1(x = L, t = 0) \tag{5.4b}$$

$$\frac{\partial u_1(x = L, t)}{\partial x} = \frac{\partial u_1(x = 0, t)}{\partial x} \tag{5.4c}$$

$$u_2(x, t = 0) = 0 \tag{5.4d}$$

where $g_s(x,t)$ is a source term added to the $u_1(x,t)$ PDE to represent the drug injection as a function of position and time. Note also that the elimination term based on $g(t)u_1$ in eq. (5.1a) has been eliminated. Thus, eq. (5.3a) includes the following phenomena and associated mathematical terms.

- Diffusion: $D_1\dfrac{\partial^2 u_1}{\partial x^2}$
- Convection: $-\dfrac{\partial[v(x,t)u_1]}{\partial x}$
- Binding: $-k_b u_1(u_2^e - u_2)$
- Injection: $g_s(x,t)$
- Accumulation (depletion): $\dfrac{\partial u_1}{\partial t}$

$g_s(x,t)$ in the following R implementation can be a function of essentially any form and therefore is a substantial generalization of the delta function in IC (5.2a). Note also that the IC for eq. (5.3a), eq. (5.4a), is now homogeneous (zero rather than a delta function), which facilitates the numerical solution. Thus, the solution that is subsequently developed for eqs. (5.3) and (5.4) is the response to only $g_s(x,t)$ in eq. (5.3a).

5.4.1 ODE Routine for the Extended Model

The MOL/ODE routines for eqs. (5.3) and (5.4) is in Listing 5.6.

```
  pharma_2=function(t,u,parms){
#
# Function pharma_2 computes the t derivative vector
# of the u1,u2 vectors
#
# One vector to two vectors
  u1=rep(0,nx);u2=rep(0,nx);
  for(i in 1:nx){
    u1[i]=u[i];
    u2[i]=u[i+nx];
  }
```

```
#
# Boundary conditions
  u1[1]=u1[nx];
  u1x=dss004(xl,xu,nx,u1);
  u1x[nx]=u1x[1];
  nl=1;nu=2;
#
# u1xx
  u1xx=dss044(xl,xu,nx,u1,u1x,nl,nu);
#
# (v*u1)x
  vu1=rep(0,nx);
  for(i in 1:nx){
    vu1[i]=vf(xg[i],t)*u1[i];
  }
# vu1x=dss004(xl,xu,nx,vu1);
  vu1x=dss012(xl,xu,nx,vu1,1);
#
# PDEs
  u1t=rep(0,nx);u2t=rep(0,nx);
  for(i in 1:nx){
    u1t[i]=D1*u1xx[i]-vu1x[i]-kb*u1[i]*(u1e-u1[i])+
       gs(xg[i],t);
    u2t[i]=kb*u1[i]*(u1e-u1[i]);
  }
  u1t[1]=0;
#
# Two vectors to one vector
  ut=rep(0,2*nx);
  for(i in 1:nx){
    ut[i]   =u1t[i];
    ut[i+nx]=u2t[i];
  }
#
# Increment calls to pharma_2
  ncall <<- ncall+1;
#
# Return derivative vector
  return(list(c(ut)));
}
```

Listing 5.6 ODE routine for eqs. (5.3), (5.4b), and (5.4c).

Listing 5.6 is similar to Listing 5.2. The only essential difference is the coding for eqs. (5.1a) and (5.3a) in which the function g_e is replaced with g_s.

```
Listing 5.2

    u1t[i]=D1*u1xx[i]-vu1x[i]-ge(t)*u1[i]-kb*u1[i]*
       (u1e-u1[i]);

Listing 5.6

    u1t[i]=D1*u1xx[i]-vu1x[i]-kb*u1[i]*(u1e-u1[i])+
       gs(xg[i],t);
```

Also, IC (5.2a) in Listing 5.1 is replaced with IC (5.4a) in Listing 5.8 to follow.

Function gs is in Listing 5.7.

```
  gs=function(x,t){
#
# Function gs computes the inhomogeneous source term
#
  g=0;
  if((t>=0)&&(t<=1)){
    if((x>0.495)&&(x<0.505)){
      g=1;
    }
  }
  return(c(g));
  }
```

Listing 5.7 Function gs for function g_s in eq. (5.3a).

We can note the following details about gs.

- The function is defined with the two input arguments x and t as required by the call to gs for eq. (5.3a).
- gs is set to zero and then redefined to 1 for $0 \leq t \leq 1$ and $0.495 > x < 0.505$. The range in x actually specifies $x = 0.5$ only because with the gridding in x, other values of x are

excluded. In other words, the value $g_s(x = 0.5, t) = 1$ is selected. This particular example illustrates the generality of $g_s(x, t)$ as a function of x and t.

- A numerical vector with one element, the value of $g_s(x, t)$, is returned to the calling program. The final `}` concludes `gs`.

Discussion of the main program for eqs. (5.3) and (5.4) is in Section 5.4.2.

5.4.2 Main Program for the Extended Model

The main program is the same as in Listing 5.1 except that IC (5.4a) is used and the ODE routine called by `lsodes` is `pharma_2` of Listing 5.6 rather than `pharma_1` of Listing 5.1.

```
#
# IC
  u0=rep(0,2*nx);
  ncall=0;
      .
      .
      .
#
# ODE integration
  out=lsodes(y=u0,times=tout,func=pharma_2,parms=NULL)
  nrow(out)
  ncol(out)
```

Listing 5.8 Partial listing of the main program for eqs. (5.3) and (5.4).

Thus, basically the call to `pharma_2` reflects the contribution of g_s in eq. (5.3a).

The numerical and graphical outputs from Listings 5.6–5.8 is considered in Section 5.4.3.

5.4.3 Output for the Extended Model

The abbreviated output from Listing 5.8 (and output as programmed in Listing 5.1) follows.

We can note the following details for the output in Table 5.3.

- For $t = 0$, ICs (5.4a) and (5.4d) are confirmed (in particular, the delta function of IC (5.2a) has been replaced with a zero for $u_1(x = 0.5, t = 0)$).
- For $t = 2$ and the values of x included, $u_1(x, t = 2)$ has departed from zero IC because of the function `gs` in Listing 5.7. Also, $u_2(x, t = 2)$ has responded to `gs`.
- For $t = 10$, $u_1(x, t = 10)$ has decayed to essentially zero and $u_2(x, t = 10)$ displays a significant bound drug concentration.
- The computational effort is modest with `ncall` $= 438$.

The features of the solution $u_1(x, t), u_2(x, t)$ are clearer from the graphical output in Fig. 5.7, which indicates the effect of $g_s(x, t)$ with peaking of $u_1(x, t)$ in the neighborhood of $x = 0.5$ followed by a decay close to $u_1(x, t = 10) = 0$ as reflected in Table 5.3. Figure 5.8 indicates that dropping the solution $u_1(x, t = 0)$ of Fig. 5.7 has no unexpected effect. This contrasts with a comparison of Figs. 5.1 and 5.2 reflecting the effect of the delta function of IC (5.2a). Figure 5.9 indicates the accumulation of the bound drug in

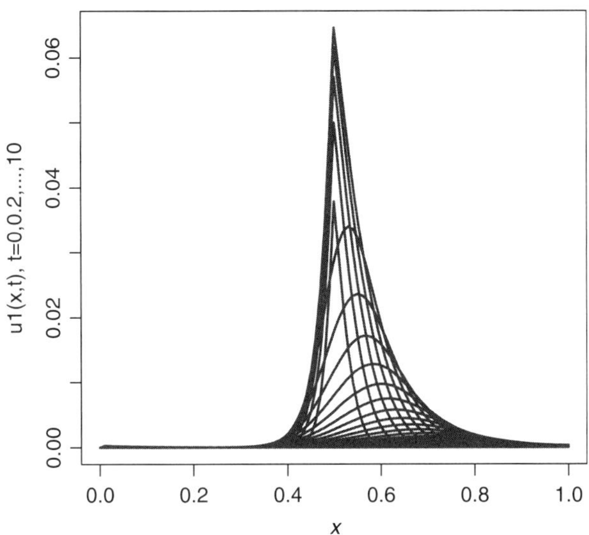

Figure 5.7 $u_1(x, t)$ versus x with t as a parameter, $t = 0, 0.2, \ldots, 10$.

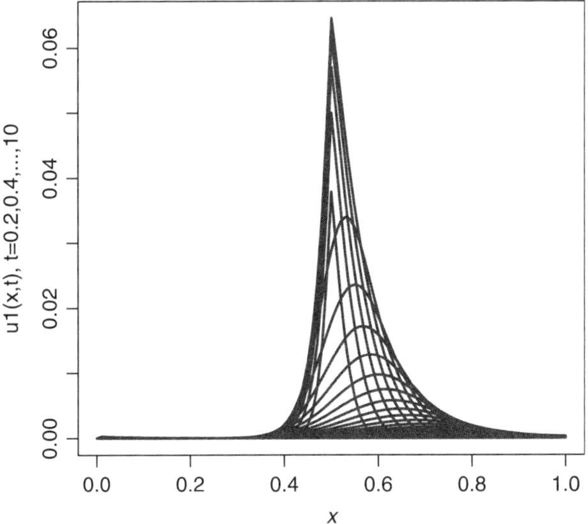

Figure 5.8 $u_1(x,t)$ versus x with t as a parameter, $t = 0.2, \ldots, 10$.

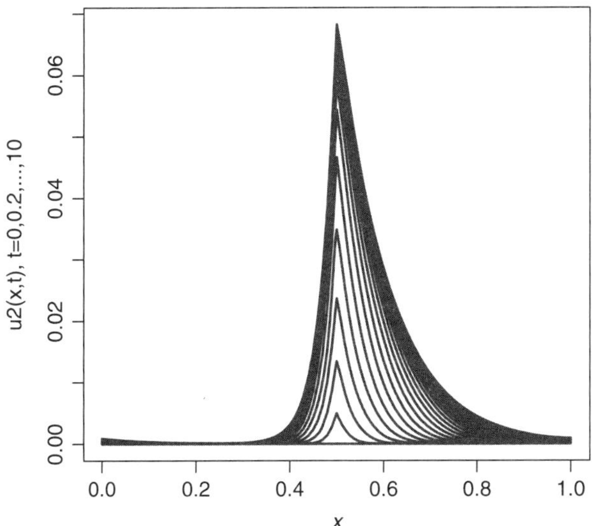

Figure 5.9 $u_2(x,t)$ versus x with t as a parameter, $t = 0, 0.2, \ldots, 10$.

TABLE 5.3 Abbreviated output from Listings 5.5–5.7.

```
D1 = 3.000e-03  kb =  1.000  u1e =  1.000
   ms =  1.000

Peclet number = 25.00

    t      x    u1(x,t)   u2(x,t)
  0.0  0.000   0.00000   0.00000
  0.0  0.010   0.00000   0.00000
  0.0  0.020   0.00000   0.00000
  0.0  0.030   0.00000   0.00000
  0.0  0.040   0.00000   0.00000
  0.0  0.050   0.00000   0.00000
         .                 .
         .                 .
         .                 .
  Output from x = 0.060 to 0.440
               removed
         .                 .
         .                 .
         .                 .
  0.0  0.450   0.00000   0.00000
  0.0  0.460   0.00000   0.00000
  0.0  0.470   0.00000   0.00000
  0.0  0.480   0.00000   0.00000
  0.0  0.490   0.00000   0.00000
  0.0  0.500   0.00000   0.00000
  0.0  0.510   0.00000   0.00000
  0.0  0.520   0.00000   0.00000
  0.0  0.530   0.00000   0.00000
  0.0  0.540   0.00000   0.00000
  0.0  0.550   0.00000   0.00000
         .                 .
         .                 .
         .                 .
  Output from x = 0.560 to 0.940
               removed
         .                 .
         .                 .
```

TABLE 5.3 (*Continued*)

```
         .                 .
 0.0  0.950   0.00000   0.00000
 0.0  0.960   0.00000   0.00000
 0.0  0.970   0.00000   0.00000
 0.0  0.980   0.00000   0.00000
 0.0  0.990   0.00000   0.00000
 0.0  1.000   0.00000   0.00000

   t      x   u1(x,t)   u2(x,t)
 2.0  0.000   0.00000   0.00000
 2.0  0.010   0.00001   0.00000
 2.0  0.020   0.00001   0.00000
 2.0  0.030   0.00001   0.00000
 2.0  0.040   0.00001   0.00000
 2.0  0.050   0.00000   0.00000
         .                 .
         .                 .
         .                 .
 Output from x = 0.060 to 0.440
                removed
         .                 .
         .                 .
         .                 .
 2.0  0.450   0.00278   0.01328
 2.0  0.460   0.00327   0.01855
 2.0  0.470   0.00380   0.02580
 2.0  0.480   0.00438   0.03572
 2.0  0.490   0.00498   0.04902
 2.0  0.500   0.00560   0.06494
 2.0  0.510   0.00623   0.06017
 2.0  0.520   0.00685   0.05457
 2.0  0.530   0.00745   0.04928
 2.0  0.540   0.00800   0.04435
 2.0  0.550   0.00850   0.03979
         .                 .
         .                 .
         .                 .
```

(*continued*)

TABLE 5.3 (*Continued*)

```
  Output from x = 0.560 to 0.940
                removed
          .                 .
          .                 .
          .                 .
  2.0  0.950    0.00005    0.00001
  2.0  0.960    0.00004    0.00001
  2.0  0.970    0.00003    0.00001
  2.0  0.980    0.00003    0.00001
  2.0  0.990    0.00002    0.00000
  2.0  1.000    0.00002    0.00000
          .                 .
          .                 .
          .                 .
  Output from t = 4 to 8 removed
          .                 .
          .                 .
          .                 .
    t       x   u1(x,t)    u2(x,t)
 10.0  0.000    0.00000    0.00089
 10.0  0.010    0.00000    0.00081
 10.0  0.020    0.00000    0.00074
 10.0  0.030    0.00000    0.00067
 10.0  0.040    0.00000    0.00061
 10.0  0.050    0.00000    0.00056
          .                 .
          .                 .
          .                 .
  Output from x = 0.060 to 0.440
                removed
          .                 .
          .                 .
          .                 .
 10.0  0.450    0.00000    0.01499
 10.0  0.460    0.00000    0.02053
 10.0  0.470    0.00000    0.02809
 10.0  0.480    0.00000    0.03832
 10.0  0.490    0.00000    0.05196
```

TABLE 5.3 *(Continued)*

```
 10.0  0.500   0.00000   0.06825
 10.0  0.510   0.00000   0.06385
 10.0  0.520   0.00000   0.05863
 10.0  0.530   0.00000   0.05372
 10.0  0.540   0.00000   0.04918
 10.0  0.550   0.00000   0.04499
          .                 .
          .                 .
          .                 .
  Output from x = 0.560 to 0.940
              removed
          .                 .
          .                 .
          .                 .
 10.0  0.950   0.00000   0.00114
 10.0  0.960   0.00000   0.00106
 10.0  0.970   0.00000   0.00099
 10.0  0.980   0.00000   0.00093
 10.0  0.990   0.00000   0.00090
 10.0  1.000   0.00000   0.00089

 ncall =   438
```

the neighborhood of $x = 0.5$ (again through the influence of $g_s(x, t)$ in eq. (5.3a)). Figure 5.10 indicates the change in $u_1(x = 0.8, t)$ as a function of t (compare this with Fig. 5.4). Figure 5.11 indicates the change in $u_2(x = 0.8, t)$ as a function of t (compare this with Fig. 5.5).

Figs. 5.12 and 5.13 are 3D plots of $u_1(x, t)$ and $u_2(x, t)$ produced by the following code added to the main program. For $u_1(x, t)$,

```
#
# u1, u2 3D color plotting
#
# Color scheme
  jet2.colors <- colorRampPalette(
```

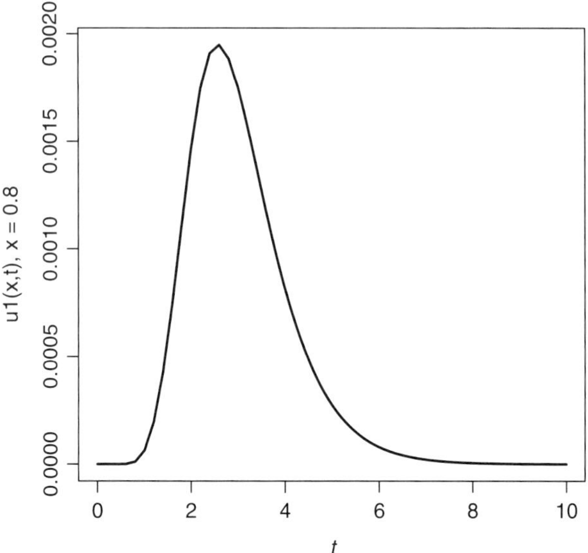

Figure 5.10 $u_1(x,t)$ versus t, $x = 0.8$.

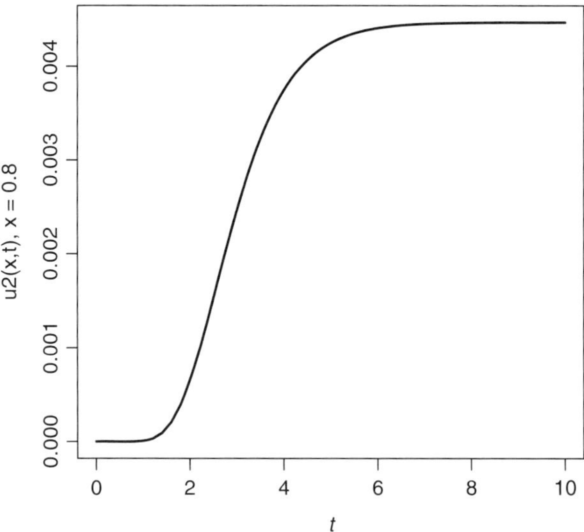

Figure 5.11 $u_2(x,t)$ vs t, $x = 0.8$

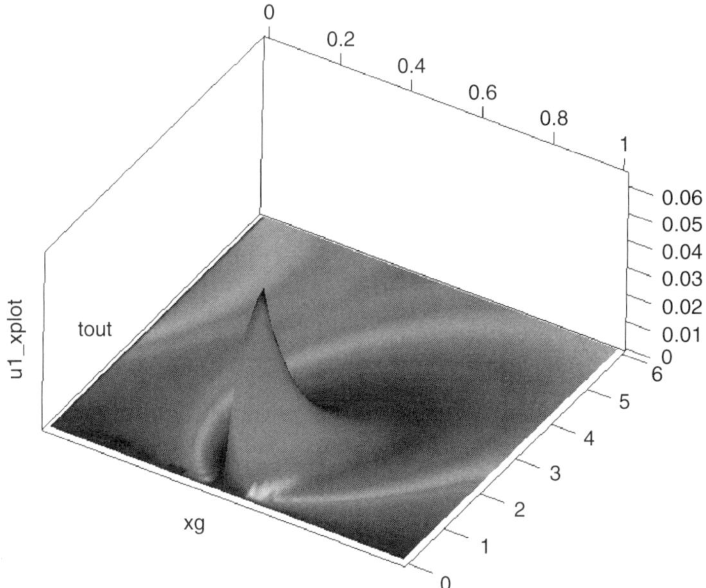

Figure 5.12 $u_1(x,t)$ versus t and x.

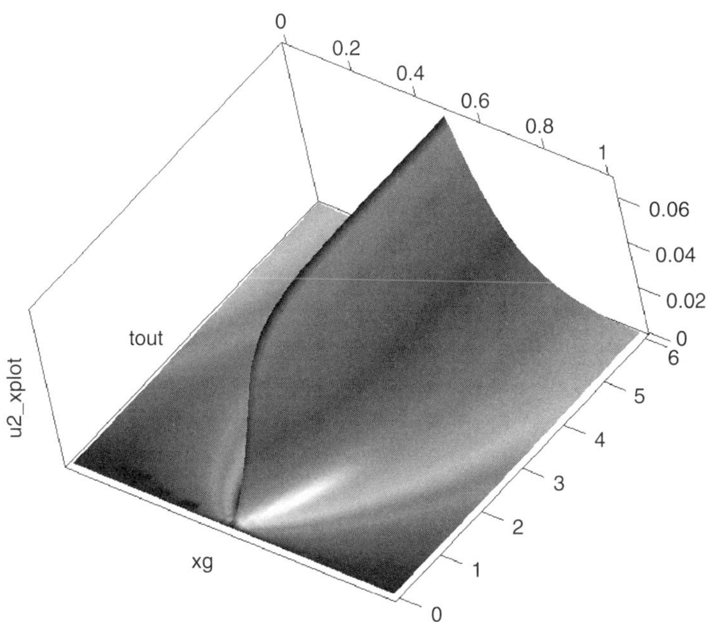

Figure 5.13 $u_2(x,t)$ versus t and x.

```
     c("black","blue","cyan","yellow","red","magenta"))
#
# Palette
  pal <- jet2.colors(length(u1_xplot))[rank(u1_xplot)]
#
# 3D plotting
  open3d()
  bg3d("white")
  persp3d(xg,tout,u1_xplot,col=pal,aspect=c(1,1,0.5),
          box=FALSE,axes=TRUE,smooth=TRUE)
#
# View point
  rgl.viewpoint(theta=-10,phi=-45,fov=0)
#
# 3D titles
  title3d(" ",at=c(0,0,1),col='red',line=3)
#
# Display parameters
  par3d(windowRect=c(20,100,820,900),zoom=1)
#
# Write to png file
# rgl.snapshot("u1(x,t).png",fmt="png")
```

This code (provided by Professor G. W. Griffiths) is not discussed here in detail. We can note the following points.

- The 3D plot can be rotated manually before being converted to a png file with `rgl.snapshot("u1(x,t).png",fmt="png")` (Fig. 5.12).
- The 3D plot for $u_2(x,t)$ (Fig. 5.13) is produced by changing `u1` to `u2` in the preceding code.
- The R graphics library `rgl` is required and is accessed with

```
#
# Access ODE integrator
  library("deSolve");
  library("rgl");
```

This completes the discussion of the extended model of eqs. (5.3) and (5.4). To recapitulate, adding the inhomogeneous source term $g_s(x,t)$ to eq. (5.3a) is straightforward and gives increased flexibility to the model (e.g., for alternative drug dosing scenarios) not provided by the delta function of eq. (5.2a).

As a final comment on the difference in the model of eqs. (5.1) and (5.2) and the model of eqs. (5.3) and (5.4), we could ask whether there is a basic difference in the use of the delta function, $u_1(x,t=0) = \delta(x-0.5)$ of IC (5.2a) and the pulse function of $g_s(x=0.5, 0 \leq t \leq 1) = 1$ in eq. (5.3a). An important difference is that the delta function pertains directly to $u_1(x,t)$ while the pulse function pertains to $u_1(x,t)$ through the derivative $\partial u_1(x,t)/\partial t$ (the LHS eq. (5.3a)). For the latter, an integration in t is required to give $u_1(x,t)$, and this integration is a smoothing process that facilitates the calculation of a numerical solution for $u_1(x,t)$. Through this reasoning, we can generally expect the use of $g_s(x,t)$ to be easier computationally than the use of the delta function.

Acknowledgment

The expert background and comments of Dr. Oscar Linares are gratefully acknowledged. The 3D plotting of $u_1(x,t), u_2(x,t)$ was generously provided by Professor G. W. Griffiths.

References

[1] Lafrance, P., V. Lemaire, F. Varin, F. Donati, and J. Belair (2002), Spatial effects in modeling pharmacokinetics of rapid action drugs, *Bull. Math. Bio.*, **64**, 483–500.

[2] Schiesser, W.E., and G.W. Griffiths (2009), *A Compendium of Partial Differential Equation Models*, Cambridge University Press, Cambridge, UK.

[3] Schiesser, W.E. (2013), *Partial Differential Equation Analysis in Biomedical Engineering*, Cambridge University Press, Cambridge, UK.

CHAPTER 6

Influenza with Vaccination and Diffusion

6.1 Introduction

The PDE model discussed in this chapter pertains to spatial and temporal effects of vaccination and diffusion in influenza epidemics [1]. The model consists of five 1D partial differential equations (PDEs with the dependent variables

1. $S(x,t)$, susceptibles
2. $V(x,t)$, vaccinated
3. $E(x,t)$, exposed
4. $I(x,t)$, infected
5. $R(x,t)$, recovered

so the model can be classified as SVEIR. x is a spatial variable to account for the spread of influenza and t is time.

The model is represented diagrammatically in Fig. 6.1 ([1], Fig. 1). The intent of the following presentation is to demonstrate:

- A system of five simultaneous (coupled) 1D PDEs programmed in R.
- Specification of no flux boundary conditions (BCs) and Gaussian function initial conditions (ICs).
- Diffusion to model the spatial spread of influenza.

Differential Equation Analysis in Biomedical Science and Engineering: Partial Differential Equation Applications with R, First Edition. William E. Schiesser.

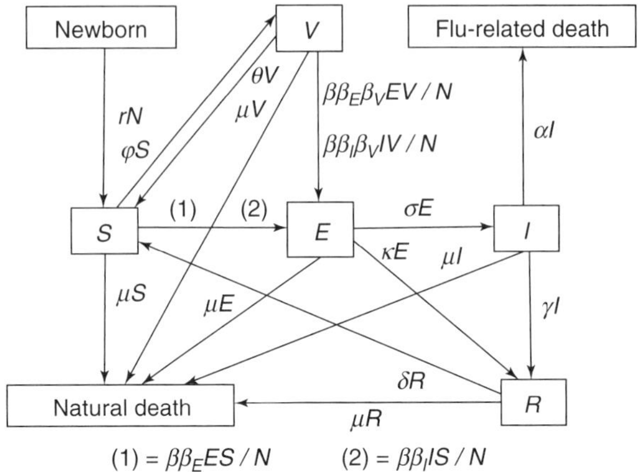

Figure 6.1 Diagram of the influenza model.

- Numerical integration of the model PDEs using the method of lines (MOL).
- A variety of numerical and graphical output formats for the five PDE solutions (dependent variables listed above).
- Rather typical challenges and uncertainties of reproducing numerical solutions to PDE models reported in the open literature.

6.2 Five PDE Model

The five PDEs of the influenza model are listed next (note in particular the five dependent variables $S(x,t), V(x,t), E(x,t), I(x,t), R(x,t)$).

$$\frac{\partial S}{\partial t} = -\beta\beta_E ES - \beta\beta_I IS + \alpha IS - \phi S - rS + \delta R$$
$$+\theta V + r + d_1 \frac{\partial^2 S}{\partial x^2} \tag{6.1a}$$

$$\frac{\partial V}{\partial t} = -\beta\beta_E\beta_V EV - \beta\beta_I\beta_V IV + \alpha IV - rV$$
$$-\theta V + \phi S + d_2 \frac{\partial^2 V}{\partial x^2} \tag{6.1b}$$

$$\frac{\partial E}{\partial t} = \beta\beta_E ES + \beta\beta_I IS + \beta\beta_E\beta_V EV + \beta\beta_I\beta_V IV + \alpha IE - (r+\kappa+\sigma)E + d_3\frac{\partial^2 E}{\partial x^2} \tag{6.1c}$$

$$\frac{\partial I}{\partial t} = \sigma E - (r+\alpha+\gamma)I + \alpha I^2 + d_4\frac{\partial^2 I}{\partial x^2} \tag{6.1d}$$

$$\frac{\partial R}{\partial t} = \kappa E + \gamma I - rR - \delta R + \alpha IR + d_5\frac{\partial^2 R}{\partial x^2} \tag{6.1e}$$

Eqs. (6.1) are second order in x and therefore require two BCs for each PDE. In this case, the following no flux (zero diffusion) BCs are used.

$$\frac{\partial S(x=-3,t)}{\partial x} = \frac{\partial S(x=3,t)}{\partial x} = 0 \tag{6.2a}$$

$$\frac{\partial V(x=-3,t)}{\partial x} = \frac{\partial V(x=3,t)}{\partial x} = 0 \tag{6.2b}$$

$$\frac{\partial E(x=-3,t)}{\partial x} = \frac{\partial E(x=3,t)}{\partial x} = 0 \tag{6.2c}$$

$$\frac{\partial I(x=-3,t)}{\partial x} = \frac{\partial I(x=3,t)}{\partial x} = 0 \tag{6.2d}$$

$$\frac{\partial R(x=-3,t)}{\partial x} = \frac{\partial R(x=3,t)}{\partial x} = 0 \tag{6.2e}$$

The interval in x has been changed from the original $-2 \le x \le 2$ in [1] to $-3 \le x \le 3$. This increase is based on the observation that the solutions did not have a zero slope at the boundaries in accordance with the BCs (eqs. (6.2)).

Eqs. (6.1) are first order in t and therefore require one IC for each PDE, which is stated subsequently as eqs. (6.3).

The parameters of eqs. (6.1) are listed in Table 6.1. The use of these parameters is elucidated by Fig. 6.1. For example, the RHS terms of eq. (6.1a) for streams coming to the S block are $+\delta R$, $+\theta V$, and $+r$ (the + indicates an increase in the LHS derivative $\partial S/\partial t$). The RHS terms of eq. (6.1a) for streams leaving the S block are $-\beta\beta_E ES$, $-\beta\beta_I IS$, $-\phi S$, and $-\mu S$ (the $-$ indicates a decrease in the LHS derivative $\partial S/\partial t$). The diffusion term $d_1\partial^2 S/\partial x^2$ can either add to or subtract from S depending on the direction of the diffusion and is not included in Fig. 6.1.

TABLE 6.1 Model parameters[a].

Parameter	Description	Value
β	contact rate	0.5140
β_E	ability to cause infection by exposed individuals ($0 \leq \beta_E \leq 1$)	0.2500
β_I	ability to cause infection by infectious individuals ($0 \leq \beta_I \leq 1$)	1
$1 - \beta_V$	factor by which the vaccine reduces infection ($0 \leq \beta_V \leq 1$)	Variable
σ^{-1}	mean duration of latency (days)	2.000
γ^{-1}	mean recovery time for clinically ill (days)	5.000
δ^{-1}	duration of immunity loss (days)	365
μ	natural mortality rate	5.500×10^{-8}
r	birth rate	7.140×10^{-5}
κ	recovery rate of latents	1.857×10^{-4}
α	flu-induced mortality rate	9.300×10^{-6}
θ^{-1}	duration of vaccine-induced immunity loss (days)	365
ϕ	rate of vaccination	Variable
d_1	diffusivity, eq. (6.1a)	0.05
d_2	diffusivity, eq. (6.1b)	0.05
d_3	diffusivity, eq. (6.1c)	0.025
d_4	diffusivity, eq. (6.1d)	0.001
d_5	diffusivity, eq. (6.1e)	0

[a]Ref. 1.

In addition, positive terms with α are included in eqs. (6.1), that is, αIS (eq. 6.1a), αIV (eq. 6.1b), αIE (eq. 6.1c), αI^2 (eq. 6.1d), and αIR (eq. 6.1e). The origin and significance of these terms are not explained in the original reference other than with the statement

"After some calculations ..." and are not included in the diagram of the PDE model ([1], Fig. 1, p 124).

In addition to the change in the spatial interval (to $-3 \le x \le 3$), the following changes and/or additions were used in the programming discussed subsequently.

- The interval in t was changed from $0 \le t \le 2000$ days to $0 \le t \le 60$ days. This reduction in the interval in t was made to gain a better resolution of the changes in the numerical solutions with x and t as discussed subsequently.
- The unassigned parameter in [1], β_V, was given the value $\beta_V = 0.9$ which is within the stated limits $0 \le \beta_V \le 1$.
- The unassigned parameter in [1], ϕ, was given the value $\phi = 0.05$. This value was selected to produce a significant variation in the solution of eqs. (6.1) with x and t. As indicated in Fig. 6.1, ϕ determines the transition of S to V (susceptibles to vaccinated) and is therefore a key parameter in determining the effect of vaccination. As the value of ϕ used in [1] was unspecified, the differences in the solutions from the present study and in [1] as discussed subsequently may be due to the difference in ϕ values.

The following details are unexplained in [1].

- The terms reflecting natural deaths, $\mu S, \mu V, \mu E, \mu I, \mu R$, included in Fig. 1 of [1], were replaced with rS, rV, rE, rI, rR in the PDEs in accordance with the original [1], which gives no explanation other than "After some calculations ..."
- The origin of the numerical values of the diffusivities d_1, d_2, d_3, d_4, d_5 used in the diffusion terms of eqs. (6.1) is unspecified.

The Gaussian IC of [1] is used in the following coding. The other ICs in [1] were not implemented to limit the volume of numerical and graphical outputs.

The five ICs in Table 6.2 are referenced as eqs. (6.3a)–(6.3e) in the subsequent discussion of the R code.

TABLE 6.2 Initial conditions for eqs. (6.1).

IC Function	Interval in x	Equation
$S(x,t=0) = 0.86\exp(-(x/1.4)^2)$	$-3 \le x \le 3$	eq. (6.3a)
$V(x,t=0) = 0.10\exp(-(x/1.4)^2)$	$-3 \le x \le 3$	eq. (6.3b)
$E(x,t=0) = 0$	$-3 \le x \le 3$	eq. (6.3c)
$I(x,t=0) = 0.04\exp(-x^2)$	$-3 \le x \le 3$	eq. (6.3d)
$R(x,t=0) = 0$	$-3 \le x \le 3$	eq. (6.3e)

6.2.1 ODE Routine

The programming of eqs. (6.1) and (6.2) as a system of approximating ODEs is in `flu_1` of Listing 6.1.

```
  flu_1=function(t,u,parms){
#
# Function flu_1 computes the t derivative vector
# of the S,V,E,I,R vectors
#
# One vector to five vectors
  S=rep(0,nx);V=rep(0,nx);
  E=rep(0,nx);I=rep(0,nx);
  R=rep(0,nx);
  for(i in 1:nx){
    S[i]=u[i];
    V[i]=u[i+nx];
    E[i]=u[i+2*nx];
    I[i]=u[i+3*nx];
    R[i]=u[i+4*nx];
  }
#
# Boundary conditions
  Sx=dss004(xl,xu,nx,S);
  Vx=dss004(xl,xu,nx,V);
  Ex=dss004(xl,xu,nx,E);
  Ix=dss004(xl,xu,nx,I);
  Rx=dss004(xl,xu,nx,R);
  Sx[1]=0;Sx[nx]=0;
  Vx[1]=0;Vx[nx]=0;
  Ex[1]=0;Ex[nx]=0;
```

```
  Ix[1]=0;Ix[nx]=0;
  Rx[1]=0;Rx[nx]=0;
  nl=2;nu=2;
#
# Sxx to Rxx
  Sxx=dss044(xl,xu,nx,S,Sx,nl,nu);
  Vxx=dss044(xl,xu,nx,V,Vx,nl,nu);
  Exx=dss044(xl,xu,nx,E,Ex,nl,nu);
  Ixx=dss044(xl,xu,nx,I,Ix,nl,nu);
  Rxx=dss044(xl,xu,nx,R,Rx,nl,nu);
#
# PDEs
  b=beta;be=betae;bi=betai;bv=betav;
  a=alpha;p=phi;d=delta;t=theta;k=kappa;
  s=sigma;g=gamma;
  St=rep(0,nx);Vt=rep(0,nx);
  Et=rep(0,nx);It=rep(0,nx);
  Rt=rep(0,nx);
  for(i in 1:nx){
    ES=E[i]*S[i];
    IS=I[i]*S[i];
    EV=E[i]*V[i];
    IV=I[i]*V[i];
    IE=I[i]*E[i];
    IR=I[i]*R[i];
    St[i]=-b*be*ES-b*bi*IS+a*IS-p*S[i]-r*S[i]
          +d*R[i]+t*V[i]+r+d1*Sxx[i];
    Vt[i]=-b*be*bv*EV-b*bi*bv*IV+a*IV-r*V[i]
          -t*V[i]+p*S[i]+d2*Vxx[i];
    Et[i]=b*be*ES+b*bi*IS+b*be*bv*EV+b*bi*bv*IV
         +a*IE-(r+k+s)*E[i]+d3*Exx[i];
    It[i]=s*E[i]-(r+a+g)*I[i]+a*I[i]^2+d4*Ixx[i];
    Rt[i]=k*E[i]+g*I[i]-r*R[i]-d*R[i]+a*IR+d5*Rxx[i];
  }
#
# Five vectors to one vector
  ut=rep(0,5*nx);
  for(i in 1:nx){
    ut[i]     =St[i];
    ut[i+nx]  =Vt[i];
    ut[i+2*nx]=Et[i];
```

```
    ut[i+3*nx]=It[i];
    ut[i+4*nx]=Rt[i];
  }
#
# Increment calls to flu_1
  ncall <<- ncall+1;
#
# Return derivative vector
  return(list(c(ut)));
}
```

Listing 6.1 ODE routine `flu_1`.

We can note the following details about Listing 6.1.

- The function is defined.

```
  flu_1=function(t,u,parms){
#
# Function flu_1 computes the t derivative vector
# of the S,V,E,I,R vectors
```

  Concerning the RHS (input) arguments of `flu_1`, `t` is the current value of t in eqs. (6.1). `u` is a $5 * 61 = 305$-vector of ODE dependent variables for the five PDE dependent variables of `S,V,E,I,R` of eqs. (6.1). `parms` for passing parameters to `flu_1` is unused.

- `u` is placed in five 61-vectors (`nx=61` is set in the main program to follow).

```
#
# One vector to five vectors
  S=rep(0,nx);V=rep(0,nx);
  E=rep(0,nx);I=rep(0,nx);
  R=rep(0,nx);
  for(i in 1:nx){
    S[i]=u[i];
    V[i]=u[i+nx];
    E[i]=u[i+2*nx];
    I[i]=u[i+3*nx];
    R[i]=u[i+4*nx];
  }
```

  The five vectors are declared (preallocated) with the `rep` utility.

- The first derivatives in x, $\partial S/\partial x$ = Sx to $\partial R/\partial x$ = Rx, are computed by the library differentiator `dss004` [2]. The input arguments to `dss004` include `xl` = -3, `xu = 3` (set in the main program).

```
#
# Boundary conditions
  Sx=dss004(xl,xu,nx,S);
  Vx=dss004(xl,xu,nx,V);
  Ex=dss004(xl,xu,nx,E);
  Ix=dss004(xl,xu,nx,I);
  Rx=dss004(xl,xu,nx,R);
  Sx[1]=0;Sx[nx]=0;
  Vx[1]=0;Vx[nx]=0;
  Ex[1]=0;Ex[nx]=0;
  Ix[1]=0;Ix[nx]=0;
  Rx[1]=0;Rx[nx]=0;
  nl=2;nu=2;
```

BCs (6.2) are then programmed with subscript `1` corresponding to $x = -3$ (the left boundary in x) and subscript `nx` corresponding to $x = 3$ (the right boundary in x). These are Neumann BCs (because the first derivatives are specified at the boundaries) which are designated with `nl=nu=2`.

- The second derivatives $\partial^2 S/\partial x^2$ = Sxx to $\partial^2 R/\partial x^2$ = Rxx are computed by `dss044`. Note the vector of first derivatives is an input to `dss044` (e.g., `Sx`) to include the BCs as well as the values of `nl,nu` to specify the Neumann BCs.

```
#
# Sxx to u5xx
  Sxx=dss044(xl,xu,nx,S,Sx,nl,nu);
  Vxx=dss044(xl,xu,nx,V,Vx,nl,nu);
  Exx=dss044(xl,xu,nx,E,Ex,nl,nu);
  Ixx=dss044(xl,xu,nx,I,Ix,nl,nu);
  Rxx=dss044(xl,xu,nx,R,Rx,nl,nu);
```

- Eqs. (6.1) are programmed. First, the parameters are redefined as single characters (e.g., `b=beta`) to simplify the programming of the PDEs. Also, vectors for the derivatives in t, for example, $\partial S/\partial t$ = St, are declared with `rep`. Then the product nonlinear terms are computed for repeated use in the programming of the PDEs, for example, $E(x,t)S(x,t)$ = ES=E[i]*S[i].

```
#
# PDEs
  b=beta;be=betae;bi=betai;bv=betav;
  a=alpha;p=phi;d=delta;t=theta;k=kappa;
  s=sigma;g=gamma;
  St=rep(0,nx);Vt=rep(0,nx);
  Et=rep(0,nx);It=rep(0,nx);
  Rt=rep(0,nx);
  for(i in 1:nx){
    ES=E[i]*S[i];
    IS=I[i]*S[i];
    EV=E[i]*V[i];
    IV=I[i]*V[i];
    IE=I[i]*E[i];
    IR=I[i]*R[i];
    St[i]=-b*be*ES-b*bi*IS+a*IS-p*S[i]-r*S[i]
          +d*R[i]+t*V[i]+r+d1*Sxx[i];
    Vt[i]=-b*be*bv*EV-b*bi*bv*IV+a*IV-r*V[i]
          -t*V[i]+p*S[i]+d2*Vxx[i];
    Et[i]=b*be*ES+b*bi*IS+b*be*bv*EV+b*bi*bv*IV
         +a*IE-(r+k+s)*E[i]+d3*Exx[i];
    It[i]=s*E[i]-(r+a+g)*I[i]+a*I[i]^2+d4*Ixx[i];
    Rt[i]=k*E[i]+g*I[i]-r*R[i]-d*R[i]+a*IR+d5*Rxx[i];
  }
```

The `for` steps along the values in x from $x = -3$ to $x = 3$. The final `}` concludes the `for`. The programming of the PDEs is essentially self-explanatory by comparison with eqs. (6.1) and demonstrates the ease of including nonlinear terms numerically.

- The five dependent derivative vectors are placed in a single derivative vector `ut` with a `for` in x for return to the ODE integrator `lsoda` (called in the main program to follow).

```
#
# Five vectors to one vector
```

```
  ut=rep(0,5*nx);
  for(i in 1:nx){
    ut[i]     =St[i];
    ut[i+nx]  =Vt[i];
    ut[i+2*nx]=Et[i];
    ut[i+3*nx]=It[i];
    ut[i+4*nx]=Rt[i];
  }
```

Note that `ut` is of length `5*nx = 5*61 = 305` that matches the length of `u` as expected. The final `}` concludes the `for`.

- The number of calls to `flu_1` is incremented and returned to the calling (main) program with `<<-`.

```
#
# Increment calls to flu_1
  ncall <<- ncall+1;
```

- The derivative vector `ut` is returned to `lsoda` as a list that is required by the R ODE integrators in the library `deSolve` (discussed next in the main program).

```
#
# Return derivative vector
  return(list(c(ut)));
}
```

The final `}` concludes `flu_1`.

This concludes the programming of the 305 ODEs that approximate eqs. (6.1). The main program that calls `flu_1` is in Listing 6.2.

6.2.2 Main Program

The main program for eqs. (6.1)–(6.3) follows.

```
#
# Access ODE integrator
  library("deSolve");
```

```
#
# Access functions for analytical solutions
  setwd("c:/R/bme_pde/chap6");
  source("flu_1.R");
  source("dss004.R");
  source("dss044.R");
#
# Format of output
#
#   ip = 1 - graphical (plotted) solutions vs x with
#            t as a parameter
#
#   ip = 2 - graphical solutions vs t at specific x
#
  ip=1;
#
# Grid in x
  nx=61;xl=-3;xu=3;
  xg=seq(from=xl,to=xu,by=(xu-xl)/(nx-1));
#
# Grid in t
  if(ip==1){nout=11;t0=0;tf=60;}
  if(ip==2){nout=61;t0=0;tf=60;}
# if(ip==2){nout=61;t0=0;tf=2000;}
  tout=seq(from=t0,to=tf,by=(tf-t0)/(nout-1));
#
# Parameters
  beta=0.5140; betae=0.250;     betai=1;      betav=0.9;
  sigma=1/2;   gamma=1/5;       delta=1/365;
                                              mu=5.50e-08;
  r=1.140e-05; kappa=1.857e-04; alpha=9.30e-06;
                                              theta=1/365;
  phi=1/20;    d1=0.05;         d2=0.05;      d3=0.025;
  d4=0.001;    d5=0;
#
# Display selected parameters
  cat(sprintf(
    "\n\n    betav = %6.3f   phi = %6.3f\n",betav,phi));
#
# ICs
  u0=rep(0,5*nx);
```

```
  for(ix in 1:nx){
    u0[ix]     =0.86*exp(-(xg[ix]/1.4)^2);
    u0[ix+nx]  =0.10*exp(-(xg[ix]/1.4)^2);
    u0[ix+2*nx]=0;
    u0[ix+3*nx]=0.04*exp(-xg[ix]^2);
    u0[ix+4*nx]=0;
  }
  ncall=0;
#
# ODE integration
  out=ode(y=u0,times=tout,func=flu_1,parms=NULL);
  nrow(out)
  ncol(out)
#
# Arrays for plotting numerical solutions
  S_xplot=matrix(0,nrow=nx,ncol=nout);
  V_xplot=matrix(0,nrow=nx,ncol=nout);
  E_xplot=matrix(0,nrow=nx,ncol=nout);
  I_xplot=matrix(0,nrow=nx,ncol=nout);
  R_xplot=matrix(0,nrow=nx,ncol=nout);
  for(it in 1:nout){
    for(ix in 1:nx){
       S_xplot[ix,it]=out[it,ix+1];
       V_xplot[ix,it]=out[it,ix+1+nx];
       E_xplot[ix,it]=out[it,ix+1+2*nx];
       I_xplot[ix,it]=out[it,ix+1+3*nx];
       R_xplot[ix,it]=out[it,ix+1+4*nx];
    }
  }
#
# Display numerical solutions (for t = 0, 60)
  if(ip==1){
  for(it in 1:nout){
    if((it-1)*(it-11)==0){
    cat(sprintf("\n\n      t      x      S(x,t)
       V(x,t)"));
    cat(sprintf("\n         E(x,t)      I(x,t)
       R(x,t)"));
      for(ix in 1:nx){
        cat(sprintf("\n %6.1f%7.2f%12.5f%12.5f",
        tout[it],xg[ix],S_xplot[ix,it],V_xplot[ix,it]));
```

```
        cat(sprintf("\n%14.5f%12.5f%12.5f",
        E_xplot[ix,it],I_xplot[ix,it],R_xplot[ix,it]));
      }
    }
    }
  }
  if(ip==2){
  for(it in 1:nout){
    if((it-1)*(it-61)==0){
    cat(sprintf("\n\n      t      x      S(x,t)
       V(x,t)"));
    cat(sprintf("\n        E(x,t)      I(x,t)
       R(x,t)"));
      for(ix in 1:nx){
        cat(sprintf("\n %6.1f%7.2f%12.5f%12.5f",
        tout[it],xg[ix],S_xplot[ix,it],V_xplot[ix,it]));
        cat(sprintf("\n%14.5f%12.5f%12.5f",
        E_xplot[ix,it],I_xplot[ix,it],R_xplot[ix,it]));
      }
    }
    }
  }
#
# Calls to ODE routine
  cat(sprintf("\n\n   ncall = %5d\n\n",ncall));
#
# Plot S,V,E,I,R numerical solutions
#
# vs x with t as a parameter, t = 0,6,...,60
  if(ip==1){
    par(mfrow=c(1,1));
    matplot(x=xg,y=S_xplot,type="l",xlab="x",
            ylab="S(x,t), t=0,6,...,60",xlim=c(xl,xu),
               lty=1,main="S(x,t); t=0,6,...,60;",lwd=2);
    par(mfrow=c(1,1));
    matplot(x=xg,y=V_xplot,type="l",xlab="x",
            ylab="V(x,t), t=0,6,...,60",xlim=c(xl,xu),
               lty=1,main="V(x,t); t=0,6,...,60;",lwd=2);
    par(mfrow=c(1,1));
    matplot(x=xg,y=E_xplot,type="l",xlab="x",
            ylab="E(x,t), t=0,6,...,60",xlim=c(xl,xu),
```

```
              lty=1,main="E(x,t); t=0,6,...,60;",lwd=2);
    par(mfrow=c(1,1));
    matplot(x=xg,y=I_xplot,type="l",xlab="x",
            ylab="I(x,t), t=0,6,...,60",xlim=c(xl,xu),
               lty=1,main="I(x,t); t=0,6,...,60;",lwd=2);
    par(mfrow=c(1,1));
    matplot(x=xg,y=R_xplot,type="l",xlab="x",
            ylab="R(x,t), t=0,6,...,60",xlim=c(xl,xu),
               lty=1,main="R(x,t); t=0,6,...,60;",lwd=2);
  }
#
# vs t at x = 0, t = 0,1,...,60
  if(ip==2){
    S_tplot=rep(0,nout);V_tplot=rep(0,nout);
    E_tplot=rep(0,nout);I_tplot=rep(0,nout);
    R_tplot=rep(0,nout);
    for(it in 1:nout){
      S_tplot[it]=S_xplot[31,it];
      V_tplot[it]=V_xplot[31,it];
      E_tplot[it]=E_xplot[31,it];
      I_tplot[it]=I_xplot[31,it];
      R_tplot[it]=R_xplot[31,it];
    }
    par(mfrow=c(1,1));
    matplot(x=tout,y=S_tplot,type="l",xlab="t",
            ylab="S(x,t), x = 0",xlim=c(t0,tf),lty=1,
            main="S(x,t); x = 0",lwd=2);
    par(mfrow=c(1,1));
    matplot(x=tout,y=V_tplot,type="l",xlab="t",
            ylab="V(x,t), x = 0",xlim=c(t0,tf),lty=1,
            main="V(x,t); x = 0",lwd=2);
    par(mfrow=c(1,1));
    matplot(x=tout,y=E_tplot,type="l",xlab="t",
            ylab="E(x,t), x = 0",xlim=c(t0,tf),lty=1,
            main="E(x,t); x = 0",lwd=2);
    par(mfrow=c(1,1));
    matplot(x=tout,y=I_tplot,type="l",xlab="t",
            ylab="I(x,t), x = 0",xlim=c(t0,tf),lty=1,
            main="I(x,t); x = 0",lwd=2);
    par(mfrow=c(1,1));
    matplot(x=tout,y=R_tplot,type="l",xlab="t",
```

```
           ylab="R(x,t), x = 0",xlim=c(t0,tf),lty=1,
           main="R(x,t); x = 0",lwd=2);
}
```

Listing 6.2 Main program for eqs. (6.1)–(6.3).

We can note the following details about this main program.

- The library of R ODE integrators, `deSolve`, is accessed (which includes `lsoda` called subsequently). Also, `flu_1` of Listing 6.1 and the two spatial differentiators `dss004`, `dss044` called in `flu_1` are accessed.

```
#
# Access ODE integrator
  library("deSolve");
#
# Access functions for analytical solutions
  setwd("c:/R/bme_pde/chap6");
  source("flu_1.R");
  source("dss004.R");
  source("dss044.R");
```

  Note the use of a forward slash / in the `setwd` (set working directory) rather than the usual backslash \.

- The format of the numerical and graphical outputs is selected.

```
#
# Format of output
#
#   ip = 1 - graphical (plotted) solutions vs x with
#            t as a parameter
#
#   ip = 2 - graphical solutions vs t at specific x
#
  ip=1;
```

  For `ip=1`, the solutions $S(x,t)$ to $R(x,t)$ are displayed as a function of x with t as a parameter with the values $t = 0, 6, \ldots, 60$

(11 values including $t = 0$). For ip=2, the solutions $S(x = 0, t)$ to $R(x = 0, t)$ are displayed for $t = 0, 1, \ldots, 60$ (61 values including $t = 0$).

- A grid in x is defined with 61 points for $-3 \leq x \leq 3$ so that xg has the spacing (3-(-3))/(61-1) = 0.1, that is, $x = -3$, $-2.9, \ldots, 3$.

```
#
# Grid in x
  nx=61;xl=-3;xu=3;
  xg=seq(from=xl,to=xu,by=(xu-xl)/(nx-1));
```

- The output values of t are defined. For ip=1, they are $t = 0, 6, \ldots, 60$, and for ip=2, $t = 0, 1, \ldots, 60$. The smaller number of points for ip=1 is used because t is a parameter in the plots of the solutions against x. The additional points for ip=2 are used to produce smooth plots in t (at $x = 0$).

```
#
# Grid in t
  if(ip==1){nout=11;t0=0;tf=60;}
  if(ip==2){nout=61;t0=0;tf=60;}
# if(ip==2){nout=61;t0=0;tf=2000;}
  tout=seq(from=t0,to=tf,by=(tf-t0)/(nout-1));
```

Also, the interval $0 \leq t \leq 2000$ is programmed for comparison of the graphical output with [1]. This case is used by activating the comment (removing #).

- The model parameters are defined numerically (and are available to flu_1 in Listing 6.1 as a consequence of a basic property of R, i.e., variables defined in a superior routine such as the main program in Listing 6.2 are available to subordinate routines such as flu_1).

```
#
# Parameters
  beta=0.5140; betae=0.250;    betai=1;  betav=0.9;
```

```
  sigma=1/2;    gamma=1/5;        delta=1/365;
                                                mu=5.50e-08;
  r=1.140e-05; kappa=1.857e-04; alpha=9.30e-06;
                                                theta=1/365;
  phi=1/20;     d1=0.05;          d2=0.05; d3=0.025;
  d4=0.001;     d5=0;
```

Note in particular the values betav=0.9, phi=1/20 that are unspecified in [1] (for β_V, ϕ in eqs. (6.1)).

- β_V, ϕ are displayed to emphasize their values.

```
#
# Display selected parameters
  cat(sprintf(
    "\n\n    betav = %6.3f   phi = %6.3f\n",betav,
       phi));
```

A line break is used here to limit the length of this coded line for printing.

- An IC vector u0 is defined with 5*nx = 5*61 = 305* elements by a for over the interval $-3 \leq x \leq 3$. This length is used to notify lsoda of the total number of ODEs to be integrated numerically.

```
#
# ICs
  u0=rep(0,5*nx);
  for(ix in 1:nx){
    u0[ix]      =0.86*exp(-(xg[ix]/1.4)^2);
    u0[ix+nx]   =0.10*exp(-(xg[ix]/1.4)^2);
    u0[ix+2*nx]=0;
    u0[ix+3*nx]=0.04*exp(-xg[ix]^2);
    u0[ix+4*nx]=0;
  }
  ncall=0;
```

The ICs for $S(x,t), V(x,t), I(x,t)$ are Gaussian functions of x specified in [1]. The counter for the calls to flu_1 is also initialized (and is available to flu_1 as a global variable).

- The 305 ODEs are integrated by `lsoda` (the default of the ODE integrator `ode`).

```
#
# ODE integration
  out=ode(y=u0,times=tout,func=flu_1,parms=NULL);
  nrow(out)
  ncol(out)
```

Note the use of the IC vector, `u0`, the vector of output values of t, `tout`, and the ODE routine `flu_1` of Listing 6.1. `y,times,func` are reserved names of `ode`. The argument for passing parameters to `flu_1`, `parms`, is unused. The number of rows and columns of the output (solution) matrix `out` are displayed to confirm the expected values. Actually, the number of columns is 306 rather than 305 because `lsoda` also returns the values of t (in addition to the 305 values of the ODE dependent variables).

- The numerical ODE solutions are placed in five 2D arrays for subsequent plotting by using the `matrix` utility.

```
#
# Arrays for plotting numerical solutions
  S_xplot=matrix(0,nrow=nx,ncol=nout);
  V_xplot=matrix(0,nrow=nx,ncol=nout);
  E_xplot=matrix(0,nrow=nx,ncol=nout);
  I_xplot=matrix(0,nrow=nx,ncol=nout);
  R_xplot=matrix(0,nrow=nx,ncol=nout);
  for(it in 1:nout){
    for(ix in 1:nx){
       S_xplot[ix,it]=out[it,ix+1];
       V_xplot[ix,it]=out[it,ix+1+nx];
       E_xplot[ix,it]=out[it,ix+1+2*nx];
       I_xplot[ix,it]=out[it,ix+1+3*nx];
       R_xplot[ix,it]=out[it,ix+1+4*nx];
    }
  }
```

Note the `for` in t with index `it` and the `for` in x with index `ix`. Also, the second argument of `out` is offset by `1` to accommodate t that is also returned by `lsoda`, for example, `ix+1`. Thus, the second index of out has the range 1 to ix+1+4*nx = 61+1+4*61 = 306 (not 305) as noted previously.

- For ip=1, the solution is displayed as a function of x (with the for in nx) and t (with the for in it).

```
#
# Display numerical solutions (for t = 0, 60)
  if(ip==1){
  for(it in 1:nout){
    if((it-1)*(it-11)==0){
    cat(sprintf("\n\n      t       x       S(x,t)
       V(x,t)"));
    cat(sprintf("\n           E(x,t)      I(x,t)
       R(x,t)"));
      for(ix in 1:nx){
        cat(sprintf("\n %6.1f%7.2f%12.5f%12.5f",
        tout[it],xg[ix],S_xplot[ix,it],V_xplot[ix,
           it]));
        cat(sprintf("\n%14.5f%12.5f%12.5f",
        E_xplot[ix,it],I_xplot[ix,it],R_xplot[ix,
           it]));
      }
    }
    }
  }
```

To limit the output to a manageable size, the solution at only $t = 0, 60$ is displayed by using if((it-1)*(it-11)==0). Of course, any of the output values of t can be selected in this way.

- The output for ip=2 is displayed in essentially the same way as for ip=1. Note again that this output is only for $t = 0, 60$ by using if((it-1)*(it-61)==0) (because there are now 61 output points in t rather than the 11 for ip=1).

```
  if(ip==2){
  for(it in 1:nout){
    if((it-1)*(it-61)==0){
    cat(sprintf("\n\n      t       x       S(x,t)
       V(x,t)"));
    cat(sprintf("\n           E(x,t)      I(x,t)
```

```
        R(x,t)"));
      for(ix in 1:nx){
        cat(sprintf("\n %6.1f%7.2f%12.5f%12.5f",
        tout[it],xg[ix],S_xplot[ix,it],V_xplot[ix,
           it]));
        cat(sprintf("\n%14.5f%12.5f%12.5f",
        E_xplot[ix,it],I_xplot[ix,it],R_xplot[ix,
           it]));
      }
    }
    }
  }
```

- The counter for the calls to `flu_1` is displayed as a measure of the effort required to compute the numerical solution.

```
#
# Calls to ODE routine
  cat(sprintf("\n\n   ncall = %5d\n\n",ncall));
```

- For `ip=1`, five individual (separate) plots for $S(x,t)$ to $R(x,t)$ are produced with `par(mfrow=c(1,1))` (a 1×1 matrix of individual plots, i.e., a single plot). Note the use of `xg` as the horizontal `x` variable and the 2D arrays with the solutions to eqs. (6.1) as the vertical `y` variable.

```
#
# Plot S,V,E,I,R numerical solutions
#
# vs x with t as a parameter, t = 0,6,...,60
  if(ip==1){
    par(mfrow=c(1,1));
    matplot(x=xg,y=S_xplot,type="l",xlab="x",
            ylab="S(x,t), t=0,6,...,60",xlim=c(xl,xu),
               lty=1,main="S(x,t); t=0,6,...,60;",
                  lwd=2);
    par(mfrow=c(1,1));
    matplot(x=xg,y=V_xplot,type="l",xlab="x",
            ylab="V(x,t), t=0,6,...,60",xlim=c(xl,xu),
               lty=1,main="V(x,t); t=0,6,...,60;",
                  lwd=2);
```

```
    par(mfrow=c(1,1));
    matplot(x=xg,y=E_xplot,type="l",xlab="x",
            ylab="E(x,t), t=0,6,...,60",xlim=c(xl,xu),
               lty=1,main="E(x,t); t=0,6,...,60;",
                  lwd=2);
    par(mfrow=c(1,1));
    matplot(x=xg,y=I_xplot,type="l",xlab="x",
            ylab="I(x,t), t=0,6,...,60",xlim=c(xl,xu),
               lty=1,main="I(x,t); t=0,6,...,60;",
                  lwd=2);
    par(mfrow=c(1,1));
    matplot(x=xg,y=R_xplot,type="l",xlab="x",
            ylab="R(x,t), t=0,6,...,60",xlim=c(xl,xu),
               lty=1,main="R(x,t); t=0,6,...,60;",
                  lwd=2);
  }
```

matplot requires that the number of rows of x equals the number of rows of y, 61 in this case. The number of columns of the y arrays is 11 (refer to the definition of the 2D y arrays discussed previously) so that t is plotted parametrically (as 11 separate curves in each plot). The other arguments of matplot pertain to labeling and line types for the plots (as reflected in Figs. 6.2–6.6).

- For ip=2, five individual plots for $S(x = 0, t)$ to $R(x = 0, t)$ are produced, again with par(mfrow=c(1,1)). The 1D arrays (vectors) for the plotting as a function of t are defined with the rep utility. The solutions for $x = 0$ are then placed in the 1D arrays (from the previous 2D arrays using subscript 31 for $x = 0$). In the calls to matplot, note the use of tout as the horizontal x variable and the 1D arrays with the solutions at $x = 0$ as the vertical y variables. The net result is the plotting of the five dependent variables from eq. (6.1) for $x = 0$ as a function of t for $t = 0, 1, \ldots, 60$. The resulting plots are in Figs. 6.7–6.11.

```
#
# vs t at x = 0, t = 0,1,...,60
  if(ip==2){
    S_tplot=rep(0,nout);V_tplot=rep(0,nout);
```

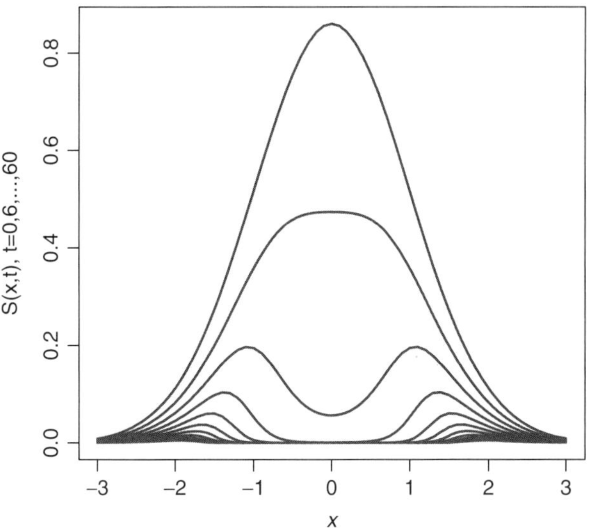

Figure 6.2 $S(x,t)$ versus x, $t = 0, 6, \ldots, 60$.

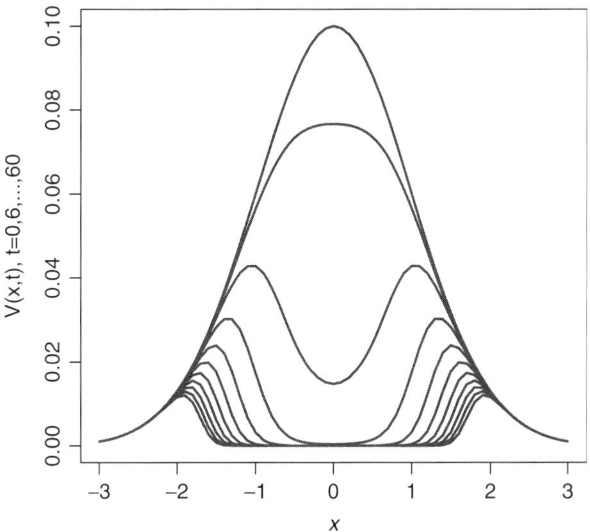

Figure 6.3 $V(x,t)$ versus x, $t = 0, 6, \ldots, 60$.

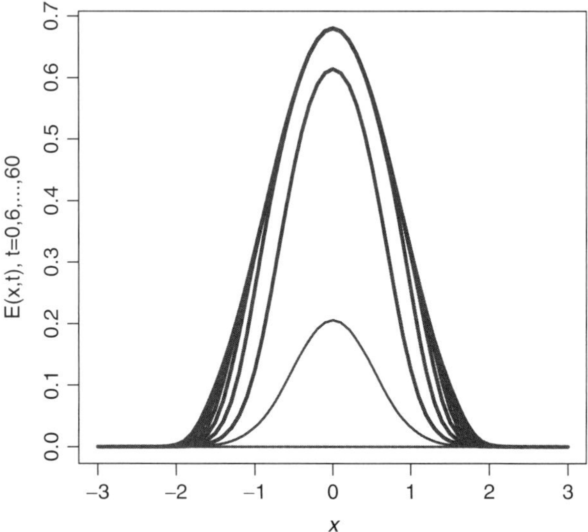

Figure 6.4 $E(x,t)$ versus x, $t = 0, 6, \ldots, 60$.

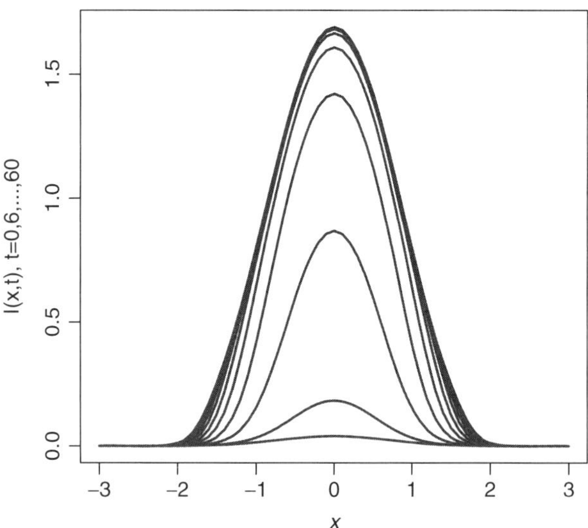

Figure 6.5 $I(x,t)$ versus x, $t = 0, 6, \ldots, 60$.

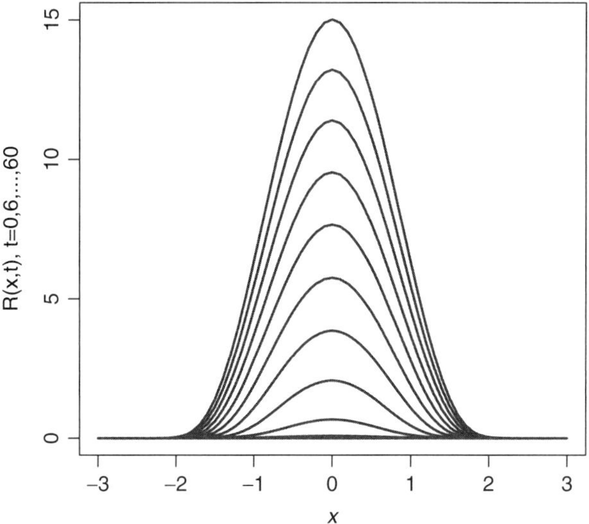

Figure 6.6 $R(x,t)$ versus x, $t = 0, 6, \ldots, 60$.

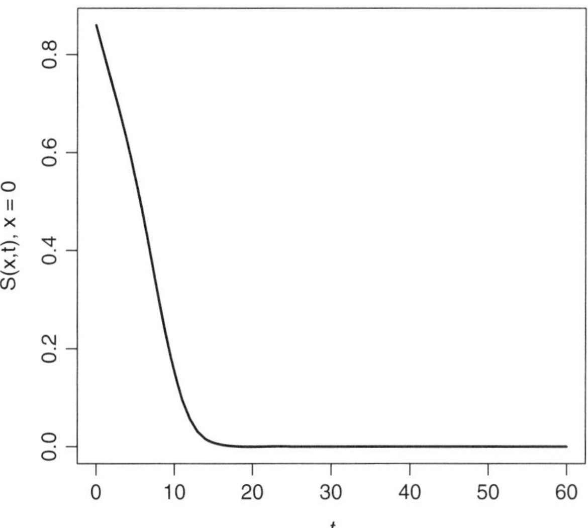

Figure 6.7 $S(x,t)$ versus t, $x = 0$.

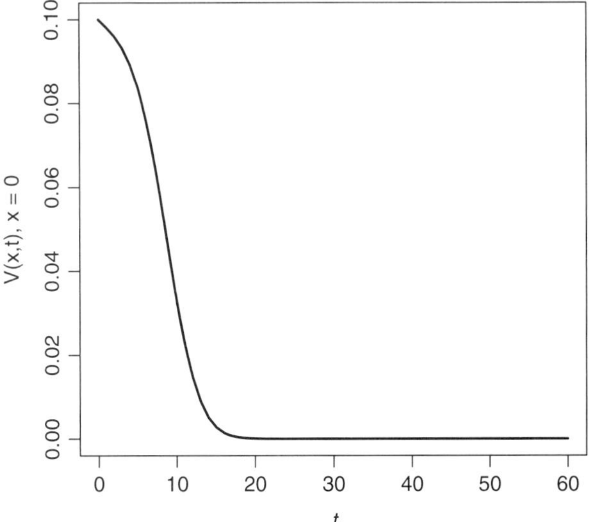

Figure 6.8 $V(x,t)$ versus t, $x = 0$.

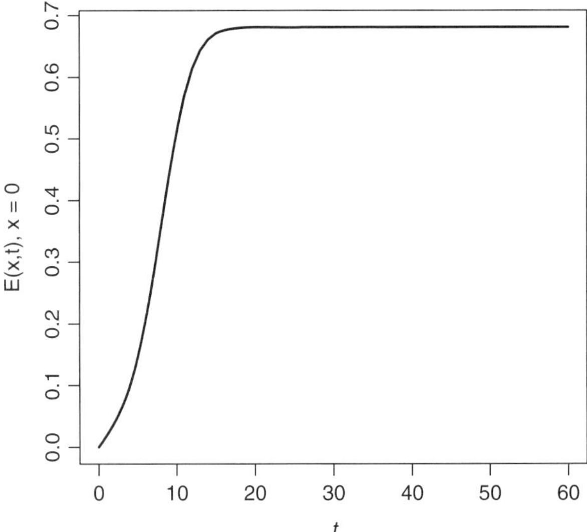

Figure 6.9 $E(x,t)$ versus t, $x = 0$.

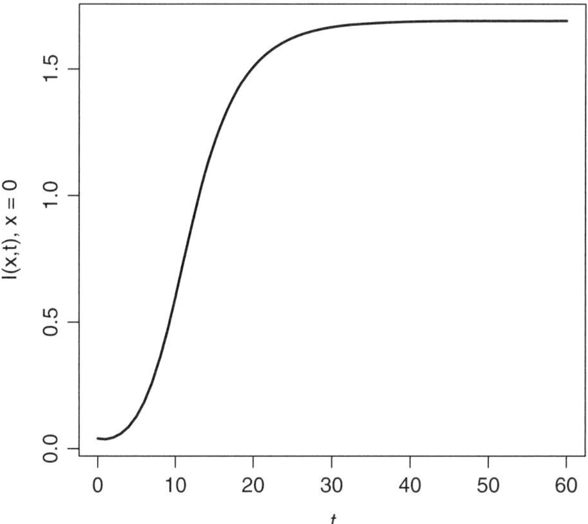

Figure 6.10 $I(x,t)$ versus t, $x = 0$.

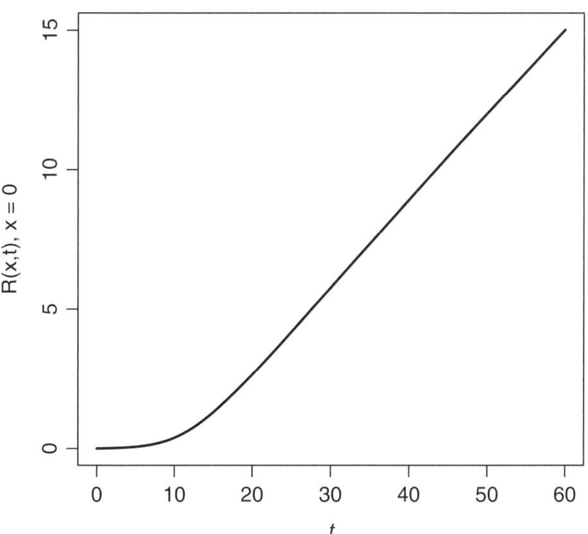

Figure 6.11 $R(x,t)$ versus t, $x = 0$.

```
    E_tplot=rep(0,nout);I_tplot=rep(0,nout);
    R_tplot=rep(0,nout);
    for(it in 1:nout){
      S_tplot[it]=S_xplot[31,it];
      V_tplot[it]=V_xplot[31,it];
      E_tplot[it]=E_xplot[31,it];
      I_tplot[it]=I_xplot[31,it];
      R_tplot[it]=R_xplot[31,it];
    }
    par(mfrow=c(1,1));
    matplot(x=tout,y=S_tplot,type="l",xlab="t",
            ylab="S(x,t), x = 0",xlim=c(t0,tf),lty=1,
            main="S(x,t); x = 0",lwd=2);
    par(mfrow=c(1,1));
    matplot(x=tout,y=V_tplot,type="l",xlab="t",
            ylab="V(x,t), x = 0",xlim=c(t0,tf),lty=1,
            main="V(x,t); x = 0",lwd=2);
    par(mfrow=c(1,1));
    matplot(x=tout,y=E_tplot,type="l",xlab="t",
            ylab="E(x,t), x = 0",xlim=c(t0,tf),lty=1,
            main="E(x,t); x = 0",lwd=2);
    par(mfrow=c(1,1));
    matplot(x=tout,y=I_tplot,type="l",xlab="t",
            ylab="I(x,t), x = 0",xlim=c(t0,tf),lty=1,
            main="I(x,t); x = 0",lwd=2);
    par(mfrow=c(1,1));
    matplot(x=tout,y=R_tplot,type="l",xlab="t",
            ylab="R(x,t), x = 0",xlim=c(t0,tf),lty=1,
            main="R(x,t); x = 0",lwd=2);
  }
```

Listings 6.1 and 6.2 produce the numerical and graphical outputs discussed in Section 6.2.3.

6.2.3 Model Output

The abbreviated numerical output from Listing 6.1 is in Table 6.3. We can note the following details about this numerical output.

- The dimensions of the output array `out` (from the ODE integrator `ode`) are

TABLE 6.3 Abbreviated numerical output from Listing 6.2 for ip=1.

```
   betav =  0.900   phi =  0.050

 [1] 11

 [1] 306

     t      x       S(x,t)      V(x,t)
          E(x,t)    I(x,t)      R(x,t)
   0.0  -3.00      0.00872     0.00101
        0.00000    0.00000     0.00000
   0.0  -2.90      0.01178     0.00137
        0.00000    0.00001     0.00000
   0.0  -2.80      0.01575     0.00183
        0.00000    0.00002     0.00000
   0.0  -2.70      0.02085     0.00242
        0.00000    0.00003     0.00000
   0.0  -2.60      0.02733     0.00318
        0.00000    0.00005     0.00000
          .                       .
          .                       .
          .                       .
 Output from x = -2.50 to -0.30 removed
          .                       .
          .                       .
          .                       .
   0.0  -0.20      0.84263     0.09798
        0.00000    0.03843     0.00000
   0.0  -0.10      0.85562     0.09949
        0.00000    0.03960     0.00000
   0.0   0.00      0.86000     0.10000
        0.00000    0.04000     0.00000
   0.0   0.10      0.85562     0.09949
        0.00000    0.03960     0.00000
   0.0   0.20      0.84263     0.09798
        0.00000    0.03843     0.00000
          .                       .
```

(continued)

TABLE 6.3 (*Continued*)

```
      .                      .
      .                      .
Output from x = 0.30 to 2.50 removed
      .                      .
      .                      .
      .                      .
  0.0    2.60     0.02733     0.00318
      0.00000     0.00005     0.00000
  0.0    2.70     0.02085     0.00242
      0.00000     0.00003     0.00000
  0.0    2.80     0.01575     0.00183
      0.00000     0.00002     0.00000
  0.0    2.90     0.01178     0.00137
      0.00000     0.00001     0.00000
  0.0    3.00     0.00872     0.00101
      0.00000     0.00000     0.00000

    t       x      S(x,t)      V(x,t)
         E(x,t)    I(x,t)      R(x,t)
 60.0   -3.00     0.00043     0.00101
      0.00000     0.00000     0.00002
 60.0   -2.90     0.00059     0.00137
      0.00000     0.00000     0.00002
 60.0   -2.80     0.00078     0.00183
      0.00000     0.00000     0.00005
 60.0   -2.70     0.00104     0.00242
      0.00000     0.00001     0.00011
 60.0   -2.60     0.00136     0.00317
      0.00001     0.00003     0.00024
      .                      .
      .                      .
      .                      .
Output from x = -2.50 to -0.30 removed
      .                      .
      .                      .
      .                      .
 60.0   -0.20    -0.00000    -0.00000
      0.66186     1.64362    14.55656
```

TABLE 6.3 (*Continued*)

```
 60.0  -0.10     -0.00000     -0.00000
      0.67593     1.67822     14.90177
 60.0   0.00     -0.00000     -0.00000
      0.68067     1.68988     15.01821
 60.0   0.10     -0.00000     -0.00000
      0.67593     1.67822     14.90177
 60.0   0.20     -0.00000     -0.00000
      0.66186     1.64362     14.55656
          .                       .
          .                       .
          .                       .
Output from x = 0.30 to 2.50 removed
          .                       .
          .                       .
          .                       .
 60.0   2.60      0.00136      0.00317
      0.00001     0.00003      0.00024
 60.0   2.70      0.00104      0.00242
      0.00000     0.00001      0.00011
 60.0   2.80      0.00078      0.00183
      0.00000     0.00000      0.00005
 60.0   2.90      0.00059      0.00137
      0.00000     0.00000      0.00002
 60.0   3.00      0.00043      0.00101
      0.00000     0.00000      0.00002

 ncall =   188
```

```
[1] 11

[1] 306
```

as expected (including `5*61 + 1` = 306 as discussed previously).

- The ICs of eqs. (6.3) (Gaussian functions in Table 6.2) can be checked approximately. For example, at $x = 0, t = 0$, the ICs are from Table 6.2 $S(x = 0, t = 0) = 0.86e^{-0^2} = 0.86$, $V(x = 0, t = 0) = 0.10$, $E(x = 0, t = 0) = 0$, $I(x = 0, t = 0) = 0.04$, $R(x = 0, t = 0) = 0$, which are confirmed in Table 6.3 as

```
    t        x          S(x,t)        V(x,t)
        E(x,t)          I(x,t)        R(x,t)

  0.0     0.00         0.86000       0.10000
        0.00000        0.04000       0.00000
```

- The ICs are symmetrical with respect to $x = 0$ as they should be from the Gaussian functions of Table 6.2 (which are even functions in x). For example,

```
    t        x          S(x,t)        V(x,t)
        E(x,t)          I(x,t)        R(x,t)

  0.0    -0.10         0.85562       0.09949
        0.00000        0.03960       0.00000
  0.0     0.00         0.86000       0.10000
        0.00000        0.04000       0.00000
  0.0     0.10         0.85562       0.09949
        0.00000        0.03960       0.00000
```

- The peak values of $S(x = 0, t = 0) = 0.86$, $V(x = 0, t = 0) = 0.10$ decrease and $E(x = 0, t)$, $I(x = 0, t = 0) = 0.04$, $R(x = 0, t)$ increase as the influenza progresses and then subsides. At $t = 60$, the values are

```
    t        x          S(x,t)        V(x,t)
        E(x,t)          I(x,t)        R(x,t)

 60.0     0.00        -0.00000      -0.00000
        0.68067        1.68988      15.01821
```

  so that $R(x, t)$ (recovered) experiences a strong increase with a significant $I(x, t)$ (infected) remaining at $t = 60$.
- The symmetry of the solutions remains as expected (there is no preferred direction in x). For example, at $t = 60$,

```
    t        x          S(x,t)        V(x,t)
        E(x,t)          I(x,t)        R(x,t)

 60.0    -0.10        -0.00000      -0.00000
```

```
         0.67593      1.67822     14.90177
  60.0     0.00      -0.00000     -0.00000
         0.68067      1.68988     15.01821
  60.0     0.10      -0.00000     -0.00000
         0.67593      1.67822     14.90177
```

which can be considered to be a check of the numerical integration of `lsoda` and the coding of the FDs in the spatial differentiators `dss004,dss044`.

The symmetry of the solutions around x is also evident in Figs. 6.2–6.6. This also suggests that the interval in x could be reduced to $0 \leq x \leq 3$ with zero derivative BCs imposed at $x = 0$ (to reflect the symmetry) rather than at $x = -3$ (to reflect zero diffusion). In other words, there is no diffusion across $x = 0$ as well as at $x = -3$.

For `ip=2`, the solutions at $x = 0$ are in Figs. 6.7–6.11. Figures 6.7–6.10 indicate that $S(x = 0, t)$ to $I(x = 0, t)$ reach steady state well before $t = 60$ while $R(x, t)$ continues to increase beyond $t = 60$. This is further confirmed by the solutions for $0 \leq t \leq 2000$ (using again `ip=2` in Listing 6.2). In Fig. 6.12, $S(x = 0, t)$ has reached steady state for $t < 60$, whereas $R(x, t)$ has reach steady state for $t < 2000$ so that the influenza has passed by $t = 2000$. In all cases, the solutions are monotonic (the LHS derivatives of eqs. (6.1) do not change sign) rather than oscillatory as reported in [1].

Figures 6.12 and 6.13 also indicate that the 305 ODE system is stiff in the sense that some of the ODEs have a fast solution, for example, $S(x = 0, t)$ in Fig. 6.12, while others have a slow solution, for example, $R(x = 0, t)$ in Fig. 6.13. It is this wide difference in the timescales that causes excessive computation when using an explicit ODE integrator. For example, $S(x = 0, t)$ requires small integration steps to maintain stability (because of the stability limit or constraint on the integration step of explicit integrators such as the explicit Euler method), while $R(x = 0, t)$ requires many steps to compute a complete solution in t.

In other words, the requirement for many small steps leads to a lengthy computation. In the case of the 305 ODE model, this

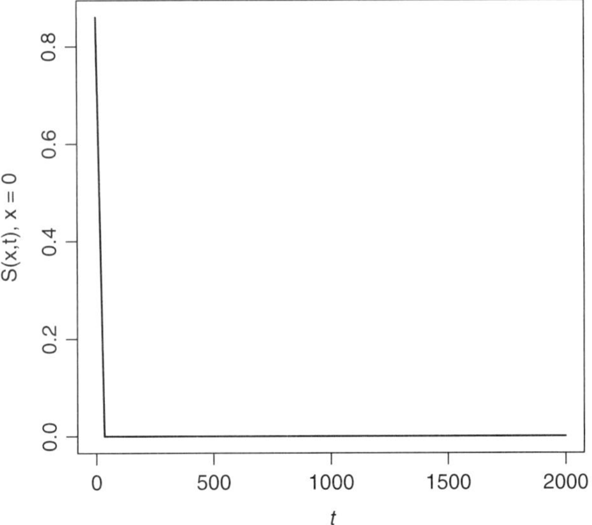

Figure 6.12 $S(x,t)$ versus t, $x = 0$.

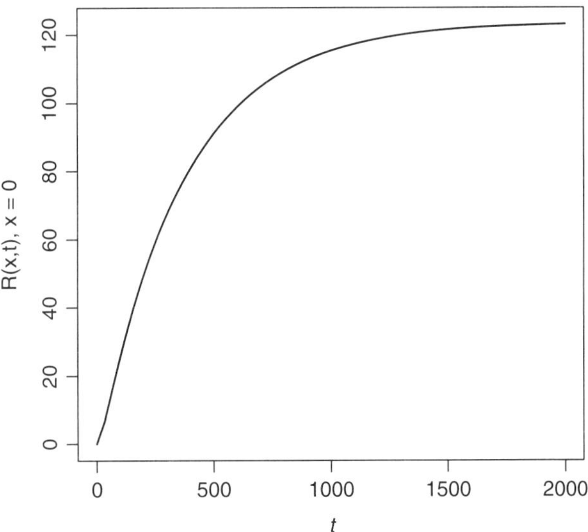

Figure 6.13 $R(x,t)$ versus t, $x = 0$.

limitation of explicit methods was circumvented by using `lsoda` in `ode` (v. Listing 6.2) that automatically switches between stiff and nonstiff methods based on an eigenvalue analysis (the "a" in `lsoda` designates the automatic switching). The effectiveness of the stiff option in lsoda is demonstrated by the modest number of calls to the ODE routine fhn_1 of Listing 6.1 such as ncall = 188 in Table 6.3.

6.3 Summary

The preceding discussion of the SVEIR model of eqs. (6.1)–(6.3) illustrates the straightforward numerical integration of a system of five 1D nonlinear PDEs. Also, this discussion illustrates the challenge of understanding the equations and reproducing the reported numerical solutions. This uncertainty in interpreting ODE/PDE models taken from the literature is not uncommon and is generally due to incomplete information such as

- Incomplete equation, IC, BC, and parameter sets.
- Reported equations with little or no indication of their origin, for example, a derivation.
- Little or no discussion of the algorithms used to compute reported numerical solutions.
- Computer codes used to compute reported numerical solutions are unavailable.

For these reasons, reproducing reported solutions is often nearly impossible. In summary, this situation of uncertainty is not unusual when accessing ODE/PDE models reported in the open literature so some additional effort and care is generally required in documenting and using the models.

References

[1] Samsuzzoha, Md., M. Singh, and D. Lucy (2012), A numerical study on an influenza epidemic model with vaccination and diffusion, *Appl. Math. Comput.*, **219**, 122–141.

[2] Schiesser, W.E., and G.W. Griffiths (2009), *A Compendium of Partial Differential Equation Models*, Cambridge University Press, Cambridge, UK.

CHAPTER 7

Drug Release Tracking

7.1 Introduction

The PDE model discussed in this chapter pertains to spatial and temporal effects in the release of a drug from a polymer matrix [1]. The principal topics of the following discussion include:

- A 3-PDE model for drug release from a polymer matrix including bound and unbound drug concentrations within the polymer matrix.
- Positive and negative effects of polymer stress on drug diffusion.
- The MOL numerical integration of the 3-PDE model.
- Comparison of stagewise and direct computation of second-order spatial derivatives for modeling the diffusion.
- Neumann and third-type (Robin, natural) BCs to model drug transfer to the environment surrounding the polymer.

Detailed discussion of the physical interpretation of the model is given in [1]. We, therefore, focus on the computational solution of the model equations.

7.2 Three PDE Model

The polymer drug delivery model consists of three 1D PDEs with the dependent variables

Differential Equation Analysis in Biomedical Science and Engineering: Partial Differential Equation Applications with R, First Edition. William E. Schiesser.

Model variable	Physical significance (for example)
$u(x,t)$	unbound drug concentration
$v(x,t)$	bound drug concentration
$\sigma(x,t)$	polymer stress

where x and t are a spatial coordinate within the polymer and time, respectively.

The three PDEs are

$$\frac{\partial u}{\partial t} = D\frac{\partial^2 u}{\partial x^2} + E\frac{\partial^2 \sigma}{\partial x^2} + f(u,v),\ -x_l \le x \le x_l,\ 0 \le t < \infty \quad (7.1a)$$

$$\frac{\partial v}{\partial t} = g(u,v),\ -x_l \le x \le x_l,\ 0 \le t < \infty \quad (7.1b)$$

$$\frac{\partial \sigma}{\partial t} + \beta\sigma = \alpha u + \gamma\frac{\partial u}{\partial t},\ -x_l \le x \le x_l,\ 0 \le t < \infty \quad (7.1c)$$

$$g(u,v) = u(u_b - u) - v(v_b - v) \quad (7.1d)$$

$$f(u,v) = -g(u,v) \quad (7.1e)$$

$D, E, \alpha, \beta, \gamma, u_b, v_b$ are constants (parameters) to be specified. The volumetric binding rates, $g(u,v)$ and $f(u,v)$ in eqs. (7.1d) and (7.1e), are expressed in terms of (nonlinear) logistic functions with limiting concentrations u_b, v_b. However, these functions can be easily modified in the following R code for any other rate functions that might be of interest.

Note also the rather unconventional diffusion term in eq. (7.1a) (and thus eq. (7.1c)) based on the stress, $E\frac{\partial^2 \sigma}{\partial x^2}$. In particular for $E > 0$, the diffusion from the conventional diffusion term $D\frac{\partial^2 u}{\partial x^2}$ (reflecting Fick's second law) is enhanced, whereas for $E < 0$, the conventional diffusion is diminished. Therefore, E is a particularly interesting parameter in this model, which is discussed subsequently in terms of some numerical solutions to eqs. (7.1).

Eqs. (7.1) are first order in t, and therefore, each requires one IC.

$$u(x,t=0)=u_0 \tag{7.2a}$$

$$v(x,t=0)=v_0 \tag{7.2b}$$

$$\sigma(x,t=0)=\sigma_0 \tag{7.2c}$$

where u_0, v_0, σ_0 are specified constants (more generally, they could be functions of x).

Eqs. (7.1a) and (7.1c) are second order in x, and therefore, each requires two BCs. For $u(x,t)$ of eq. (7.1a), the following are possibilities.

$$u(x=-x_l,t)=f_1(t) \tag{7.3a}$$

$$u(x=x_l,t)=f_2(t) \tag{7.3b}$$

$$\frac{\partial u(x=-x_l,t)}{\partial x}=f_3(t) \tag{7.3c}$$

$$\frac{\partial u(x=x_l,t)}{\partial x}=f_4(t) \tag{7.3d}$$

$$D\frac{\partial u(x=-x_l,t)}{\partial x}=-k(u_a-u(x=-x_l,t)) \tag{7.3e}$$

$$D\frac{\partial u(x=x_l,t)}{\partial x}=k(u_a-u(x=x_l,t)) \tag{7.3f}$$

where $f_1(t), f_2(t), f_3(t), f_4(t)$ are functions to be specified (time dependent BCs). Equations (7.3a) and (7.3b) are Dirichlet BCs because the dependent variable $u(x,t)$ is specified at the boundaries $x=-x_l, x_l$. Equations (7.3c) and (7.3d) are Neumann because the first derivatives of $u(x,t)$ in x are specified. Equations (7.3e) and (7.3f) are third-type (Robin, natural) BCs because both the dependent variable and its derivative are specified.

In eqs. (7.3e) and (7.3f), k is the mass transfer coefficient and u_a is the ambient concentration of the drug $u(x,t)$ in the environment surrounding the polymer. Note in particular that u_a could be a function of t, and more generally a function of spatial coordinates if the ambient concentration varies in both space of time. In this case, one or more additional PDEs would also be used to model the ambient conditions.

The second partial derivative in σ in eq. (7.1a) (and thus eq. (7.1c)) requires two BCs that are taken as homogeneous (zero) Dirichlet (eqs. (7.3g,h)) or Neumann (eqs. (7.3i,j)). In the subsequent programming, eqs. (7.3i,j) are used for $\sigma(x,t)$.

$$\sigma(x = -x_l, t) = \sigma(x = x_l, t) = 0 \tag{7.3g,h}$$

$$\frac{\partial \sigma(x = -x_l, t)}{\partial x} = \frac{\partial \sigma(x = x_l, t)}{\partial x} = 0 \tag{7.3i,j}$$

The third-type BCs of eqs. (7.3e,f) are used for $u(x,t)$.

This completes the specification of the model equations. The solutions to these equations, $u(x,t), v(x,t), \sigma(x,t)$ in numerical form, are computed by the MOL in which the derivatives in x in eqs. (7.1) are replaced by algebraic approximations (FDs). As x then does not appear explicitly in the resulting equations, only t remains as an independent variable. Thus, the approximating equations are ODEs in t that are integrated numerically by a library ODE integrator. This procedure is the essence of the MOL.

We now consider the programming of eqs. (7.1)–(7.3), starting with an ODE routine for the MOL.

7.2.1 ODE Routine

A MOL/ODE routine for eqs. (7.1) and (7.3) is listed next.

```
  drug_1=function(t,U,parms){
#
# Function drug_1 computes the t derivative vector
# of the u,v,s vectors
#
# One vector to three vectors
  u=rep(0,nx);v=rep(0,nx);
  s=rep(0,nx);
  for(i in 1:nx){
    u[i]=U[i];
```

```
    v[i]=U[i+nx];
    s[i]=U[i+2*nx];
  }
#
# ux, sx
  ux=dss004(xl,xu,nx,u);
  sx=dss004(xl,xu,nx,s);
#
# Boundary conditions
  ux[1]=-(kr/D)*(ua-u[1]);
  ux[nx]=(kr/D)*(ua-u[nx]);
  sx[1]=0;sx[nx]=0;
#
# uxx, sxx
  uxx=dss004(xl,xu,nx,ux);
  sxx=dss004(xl,xu,nx,sx);
#
# PDEs
  ut=rep(0,nx);vt=rep(0,nx)
  st=rep(0,nx);
  for(i in 1:nx){
    ut[i]=D*uxx[i]+E*sxx[i]+f_u(ub,vb,u[i],v[i]);
    vt[i]=g_v(ub,vb,u[i],v[i]);
    st[i]=alpha*u[i]-beta*s[i]+gamma*ut[i];
  }
#
# Three vectors to one vector
  Ut=rep(0,3*nx);
  for(i in 1:nx){
    Ut[i]     =ut[i];
    Ut[i+nx]  =vt[i];
    Ut[i+2*nx]=st[i];
  }
#
# Increment calls to drug_1
  ncall <<- ncall+1;
#
# Return derivative vector
  return(list(c(Ut)));
}
```

Listing 7.1 ODE routine drug_1 for eqs. (7.1) and (7.3).

We can note the following details about drug_1.

- The function is defined.

```
  drug_1=function(t,U,parms){
#
# Function drug_1 computes the t derivative vector
# of the u,v,s vectors
```

- The input dependent vector of length 3*nx = 3*51 = 153, U, is placed in three vectors, u,v,s, to facilitate the programming of eqs. (7.1).

```
#
# One vector to three vectors
  u=rep(0,nx);v=rep(0,nx);
  s=rep(0,nx);
  for(i in 1:nx){
    u[i]=U[i];
    v[i]=U[i+nx];
    s[i]=U[i+2*nx];
  }
```

  nx is defined numerically in the main program in Section 7.2.3 and is available to drug_1 as a global or shared variable. This illustrates a basic feature of R, that is, variables defined in a superior routine such as the main program are available in subordinate routines, in this case, drug_1. Also, arrays u,v,s are declared (preallocated) with the rep utility before they are used. Finally, note that the input vector of dependent variables is capital U, whereas the dependent variable for eq. (7.1a) is lower case u. In other words, we have made use of the property that R is case sensitive.

- The first derivatives, $\partial u/\partial x$, and $\partial \sigma/\partial x$, are computed by dss004.

```
#
# ux, sx
  ux=dss004(xl,xu,nx,u);
  sx=dss004(xl,xu,nx,s);
```

The boundary values of x, xl=-0.5,xu=0.5, are set in the main program. Note in particular that the calls to dss004 define the arrays ux,sx. That is, they do not have to be declared explicitly (using, e.g., rep).

- The third-type BCs of eqs. (7.3e) and (7.3f) for $u(x,t)$ and the homogeneous Neumann BCs of eqs. (7.3i) and (7.3j) for $\sigma(x,t)$ are programmed based on the arrays ux,sx defined by the previous calls to dss004.

```
#
# Boundary conditions
  ux[1]=-(kr/D)*(ua-u[1]);
  ux[nx]=(kr/D)*(ua-u[nx]);
  sx[1]=0;sx[nx]=0;
```

Again, kr,D,ua are shared between the main program and drug_1.

- The second derivatives, $\partial^2 u/\partial x^2$ and $\partial^2 \sigma/\partial x^2$, are computed by a second call to dss004.

```
#
# uxx, sxx
  uxx=dss004(xl,xu,nx,ux);
  sxx=dss004(xl,xu,nx,sx);
```

Stagewise differentiation, that is, the derivative of a derivative, is used to produce the second derivatives.

- The PDEs, eqs. (7.1), are programmed in a for after the derivatives in t are declared as arrays (with rep). Execution of the for produces 3*51 = 153 derivatives in t.

```
#
# PDEs
  ut=rep(0,nx);vt=rep(0,nx)
  st=rep(0,nx);
  for(i in 1:nx){
    ut[i]=D*uxx[i]+E*sxx[i]+f_u(ub,vb,u[i],v[i]);
    vt[i]=g_v(ub,vb,u[i],v[i]);
    st[i]=alpha*u[i]-beta*s[i]+gamma*ut[i];
  }
```

Note in particular the close correspondence of this coding with the PDEs, an important feature of the MOL. E, α, β, γ are available from the main program. Also, the binding rate functions of eqs. (7.1d,e), $f(u, v), g(u, v)$, are called as functions `f_u,g_v` discussed subsequently.

- The three derivative vectors `ut,vt,st` are placed in a single vector `Ut` to be returned to the ODE integrator called in the main program.

```
#
# Three vectors to one vector
  Ut=rep(0,3*nx);
  for(i in 1:nx){
    Ut[i]     =ut[i];
    Ut[i+nx]  =vt[i];
    Ut[i+2*nx]=st[i];
  }
```

Again, we have made use of the case-sensitive property of R to distinguish between `u` and `Ut`.

- The counter for the calls to `drug_1` is incremented and returned to the main program with `<<-`.

```
#
# Increment calls to drug_1
  ncall <<- ncall+1;
```

- The derivative vector `Ut` is returned to the ODE integrator as a list as required by the ODE integrators in the R library `deSolve`.

```
#
# Return derivative vector
  return(list(c(Ut)));
}
```

The final `}` concludes `drug_1`.

The functions `f_u,g_v` are listed in Section 7.2.2, followed by the main program (Section 7.2.3).

7.2.2 Rate Functions

The binding rate functions of eqs. (7.1d,e) called by drug_1 are straightforward (Listing 7.2).

```
  f_u=function(ub,vb,u,v){
#
# Function f_u computes the rate of binding/unbinding
#    for u
#
# Return rate function
  return(c(-u*(ub-u)+v*(vb-v)));
}

  g_v=function(ub,vb,u,v){
#
# Function g_v computes the rate of binding/unbinding
#    for v
#
# Return rate function
  return(c(u*(ub-u)-v*(vb-v)));
}
```

Listing 7.2 Functions *f(u,v),g(u,v)* of eqs. (7.1d,e)

In both f_u, g_v, the rate of binding from $u(x,t)$ to $v(x,t)$ is the logistic function u*(ub-u) and the rate of debinding from $v(x,t)$ to $u(x,t)$ is v*(vb-v). The net rate returned as a 1-vector (scalar) is then the difference of these logistic functions.

The main program that calls drug_1 is listed next.

7.2.3 Main Program

The main program that sets the model parameters and the ICs of the 153 ODEs is in Listing 7.3.

```
#
# Access ODE integrator
  library("deSolve");
#
# Access functions for analytical solutions
```

```
  setwd("c:/R/bme_pde/chap7");
  source("drug_1.R");
  source("drug_2.R");
  source("f_u.R");
  source("g_v.R");
  source("dss004.R");
  source("dss044.R");
#
# Format of output
#
#   ip = 1 - graphical (plotted) solutions vs x with
#            t as a parameter
#
#   ip = 2 - graphical solutions vs t at specific x
#
  ip=1;
#
# Select ODE routine
#
#   ncase = 1 - stagewise differentiation
#
#   ncase = 2 - direct second derivative
#
  ncase=1;
#
# Grid in x
  nx=26;xl=-0.5;xu=0.5;
  xg=seq(from=xl,to=xu,by=(xu-xl)/(nx-1));
#
# Grid in t
  if(ip==1){nout= 6;t0=0;tf=2;}
  if(ip==2){nout=41;t0=0;tf=2;}
  tout=seq(from=t0,to=tf,by=(tf-t0)/(nout-1));
#
# Parameters
  alpha=0.2; beta=1; gamma=1; D=0.6; E=0.2; kr=1;
  ub=1;      vb=1;   ua=0;
#
# Display selected parameters
  cat(sprintf(
    "\n\n    D = %6.3f    E = %6.3f\n",D,E));
```

```
#
# IC
  u0=rep(0,3*nx);
  for(ix in 1:nx){
    u0[ix]     =0.75;
    u0[ix+nx]  =0.25;
    u0[ix+2*nx]=0;
  }
  ncall=0;
#
# ODE integration
  if(ncase==1){
    out=ode(y=u0,times=tout,func=drug_1,parms=NULL);}
  if(ncase==2){
    out=ode(y=u0,times=tout,func=drug_2,parms=NULL);}
  nrow(out)
  ncol(out)
#
# Arrays for plotting numerical solutions
  u_xplot=matrix(0,nrow=nx,ncol=nout);
  v_xplot=matrix(0,nrow=nx,ncol=nout);
  s_xplot=matrix(0,nrow=nx,ncol=nout);
  for(it in 1:nout){
    for(ix in 1:nx){
       u_xplot[ix,it]=out[it,ix+1];
       v_xplot[ix,it]=out[it,ix+1+nx];
       s_xplot[ix,it]=out[it,ix+1+2*nx];
    }
  }
#
# Display numerical solutions (for t = 0,2)
  if(ip==1){
  for(it in 1:nout){
    if((it-1)*(it-6)==0){
    cat(sprintf(
      "\n\n      t       x       u(x,t)      v(x,t)
         s(x,t)"));
      for(ix in 1:nx){
        cat(sprintf("\n %6.1f%7.2f%12.5f%12.5f%12.5f",
        tout[it],xg[ix],u_xplot[ix,it],v_xplot[ix,it],
           s_xplot[ix,it]));
```

```
      }
    }
    }
  }
  if(ip==2){
  for(it in 1:nout){
    if((it-1)*(it-41)==0){
    cat(sprintf(
      "\n\n      t       x       u(x,t)       v(x,t)
         s(x,t)"));
      for(ix in 1:nx){
        cat(sprintf("\n %6.1f%7.2f%12.5f%12.5f%12.5f",
        tout[it],xg[ix],u_xplot[ix,it],v_xplot[ix,it],
           s_xplot[ix,it]));
      }
    }
    }
  }
#
# Calls to ODE routine
  cat(sprintf("\n\n   ncall = %5d\n\n",ncall));
#
# Plot u,v,s numerical solutions
#
# vs x with t as a parameter, t = 0,0.4,...,2
  if(ip==1){
    par(mfrow=c(1,1));
    matplot(x=xg,y=u_xplot,type="l",xlab="x",
            ylab="u(x,t), t=0,0.4,...,2",xlim=c(xl,xu),
               lty=1,main="u(x,t); t=0,0.4,...,2;",lwd=2);
    par(mfrow=c(1,1));
    matplot(x=xg,y=v_xplot,type="l",xlab="x",
            ylab="v(x,t), t=0,0.4,...,2",xlim=c(xl,xu),
               lty=1,main="v(x,t); t=0,0.4,...,2;",lwd=2);
    par(mfrow=c(1,1));
    matplot(x=xg,y=s_xplot,type="l",xlab="x",
            ylab="s(x,t), t=0,0.4,...,2",xlim=c(xl,xu),
               lty=1,main="s(x,t); t=0,0.4,...,2;",lwd=2);
  }
#
```

```
# vs t at x = 0, t = 0,0.05,...,2
  if(ip==2){
    u_tplot=rep(0,nout);v_tplot=rep(0,nout);
    s_tplot=rep(0,nout);
    for(it in 1:nout){
      u_tplot[it]=u_xplot[13,it];
      v_tplot[it]=v_xplot[13,it];
      s_tplot[it]=s_xplot[13,it];
     }
    par(mfrow=c(1,1));
    matplot(x=tout,y=u_tplot,type="l",xlab="t",
            ylab="u(x,t), x = 0",xlim=c(t0,tf),lty=1,
            main="u(x,t); x = 0",lwd=2);
    par(mfrow=c(1,1));
    matplot(x=tout,y=v_tplot,type="l",xlab="t",
            ylab="v(x,t), x = 0",xlim=c(t0,tf),lty=1,
            main="v(x,t); x = 0",lwd=2);
    par(mfrow=c(1,1));
    matplot(x=tout,y=s_tplot,type="l",xlab="t",
            ylab="s(x,t), x = 0",xlim=c(t0,tf),lty=1,
            main="s(x,t); x = 0",lwd=2);
  }
```

Listing 7.3 Main program for eqs. (7.1)–(7.3).

We can note the following details about Listing 7.3.

- The R ODE library `deSolve` and a series of functions are accessed. `drug_2` is a second ODE routine discussed subsequently.

```
#
# Access ODE integrator
  library("deSolve");
#
# Access functions for analytical solutions
  setwd("c:/R/bme_pde/chap7");
  source("drug_1.R");
```

```
source("drug_2.R");
source("f_u.R");
source("g_v.R");
source("dss004.R");
source("dss044.R");
```

- The form of the graphical output is specified with ip. For ip=1, the numerical solutions to eqs. (7.1), $u(x,t), v(x,t), \sigma(x,t)$, are plotted as a function of x with t as a parameter. For ip=2, the solutions are plotted as a function of t for $x = 0$.

```
#
# Format of output
#
#   ip = 1 - graphical (plotted) solutions vs x with
#            t as a parameter
#
#   ip = 2 - graphical solutions vs t at specific x
#
  ip=1;
```

- An ODE routine is selected. For ncase=1, drug_1 of Listing 7.1 is used by the ODE integrator (discussed in the following tect). For ncase=2, drug_2 is used. The difference in these routines is discussed subsequently.

```
#
# Select ODE routine
#
#   ncase = 1 - stagewise differentiation
#
#   ncase = 2 - direct second derivative
#
  ncase=1;
```

- A grid in x of nx=26 points is defined for the interval $x_l \leq x \leq x_u$, that is, $-0.5 \leq x \leq 0.5$.

```
#
# Grid in x
```

```
  nx=26;xl=-0.5;xu=0.5;
  xg=seq(from=xl,to=xu,by=(xu-xl)/(nx-1));
```

In other words, the MOL solution is computed with a spacing in x of $(0.5 - (-0.5))/(26 - 1) = 0.04$ so that $x = -0.5, -0.46, \ldots, 0.5$.

- A grid in t is defined for $0 \leq t \leq 2$. For `ip=1`, `6` output points in t are used corresponding to $t = 0, 0.4, \ldots, 2$ (the PDE solutions are plotted at $x = -0.5, -0.46, \ldots, 0.5$ with t as a parameter). For `ip=2`, `41` output points in t are used corresponding to $t = 0, 0.05, \ldots, 2$ (to produce solution plots as a function of t with $x = 0$).

```
#
# Grid in t
  if(ip==1){nout= 6;t0=0;tf=2;}
  if(ip==2){nout=41;t0=0;tf=2;}
  tout=seq(from=t0,to=tf,by=(tf-t0)/(nout-1));
```

- The model parameters, including some from [1], are defined numerically. Then the diffusivities D, E are displayed.

```
#
# Parameters
  alpha=0.2; beta=1; gamma=1; D=0.6; E=0.2; kr=1;
  ub=1;      vb=1;   ua=0;
#
# Display selected parameters
  cat(sprintf(
    "\n\n    D = %6.3f    E = %6.3f\n",D,E));
```

- The ICs of eqs. (7.2) are from [1].

```
#
# IC
  u0=rep(0,3*nx);
  for(ix in 1:nx){
    u0[ix]     =0.75;
    u0[ix+nx]  =0.25;
```

```
    u0[ix+2*nx]=0;
  }
  ncall=0;
```

Note that the ICs are placed in an IC vector `u0`. The length of this vector (`3*nx = 3*51 = 153`) specifies the number of ODEs to be integrated. Finally, the counter for the calls to `drug_1` is initialized.

- The MOL/ODEs are integrated by a call to `ode`. Note the use of `drug_1` for `ncase=1` and `drug_2` for `ncase=2`.

```
#
# ODE integration
  if(ncase==1){
    out=ode(y=u0,times=tout,func=drug_1,parms=NULL);}
  if(ncase==2){
    out=ode(y=u0,times=tout,func=drug_2,parms=NULL);}
  nrow(out)
  ncol(out)
```

The inputs to `ode` are the IC vector, `u0` (which informs `ode` of the number of ODEs), the vector of output values of t, `tout`, and the ODE routine. `y,times,func` are reserved names. `parms` for passing parameters to the ODE routine is unused. The dimensions of the solution array `out` returned by `ode` are displayed as a check on the coding.

- The solutions to eqs. (7.1) are placed in 2D arrays for subsequent plotting. These arrays are first declared with the `matrix` utility.

```
#
# Arrays for plotting numerical solutions
  u_xplot=matrix(0,nrow=nx,ncol=nout);
  v_xplot=matrix(0,nrow=nx,ncol=nout);
  s_xplot=matrix(0,nrow=nx,ncol=nout);
  for(it in 1:nout){
    for(ix in 1:nx){
       u_xplot[ix,it]=out[it,ix+1];
       v_xplot[ix,it]=out[it,ix+1+nx];
```

```
      s_xplot[ix,it]=out[it,ix+1+2*nx];
    }
  }
```

The subscripts for the 2D arrays, `ix,it`, refer to specific values of x and t. The offset of `1` in placing `out` in these arrays, for example, `ix+1`, is required because the first position in `out` is for the values of t. That is, the ODE solutions start from the second position in `out`.

- For `ip=1`, the solutions are displayed as a function of x at $t = 0, 2$ (`it=1,6`). Just these two values of t are used to conserve space in the displayed output. The IC can be checked (`it=1`) and the final solution (`it=6`) can be observed.

```
#
# Display numerical solutions (for t = 0,2)
  if(ip==1){
  for(it in 1:nout){
    if((it-1)*(it-6)==0){
    cat(sprintf(
      "\n\n     t      x      u(x,t)      v(x,t)
         s(x,t)"));
      for(ix in 1:nx){
        cat(sprintf("\n %6.1f%7.2f%12.5f%12.5f%12.5f",
        tout[it],xg[ix],u_xplot[ix,it],v_xplot[ix,it],
           s_xplot[ix,it]));
      }
    }
    }
  }
```

- For `ip=2`, the solutions are displayed as a function of x, also at $t = 0, 2$ (`it=1,41`).

```
  if(ip==2){
  for(it in 1:nout){
    if((it-1)*(it-41)==0){
    cat(sprintf(
      "\n\n     t      x      u(x,t)      v(x,t)
         s(x,t)"));
```

```
        for(ix in 1:nx){
          cat(sprintf("\n %6.1f%7.2f%12.5f%12.5f%12.5f",
          tout[it],xg[ix],u_xplot[ix,it],v_xplot[ix,it],
             s_xplot[ix,it]));
        }
      }
      }
    }
```

The difference in the range of `it` comes from the definition of the grid in t discussed previously (additional output points in t are used with `ip=2`).

- The number of calls to `drug_1` is displayed at the end of the solution as an indication of the computational required to produce the solution.

```
#
# Calls to ODE routine
  cat(sprintf("\n\n   ncall = %5d\n\n",ncall));
```

- For `ip=1`, three plots for $u(x,t)$, $v(x,t)$, $\sigma(x,t)$ are produced with `matplot`. `par(mfrow=c(1,1))` specifies a 1×1 array of plots, that is, a single plot. Note the use of the grid in x, vector `xg`, as the x (horizontal) variable.

```
#
# Plot u,v,s numerical solutions
#
# vs x with t as a parameter, t = 0,0.4,...,2
  if(ip==1){
    par(mfrow=c(1,1));
    matplot(x=xg,y=u_xplot,type="l",xlab="x",
            ylab="u(x,t), t=0,0.4,...,2",xlim=c(xl,xu),
               lty=1,main="u(x,t); t=0,0.4,...,2;",
                  lwd=2);
    par(mfrow=c(1,1));
    matplot(x=xg,y=v_xplot,type="l",xlab="x",
            ylab="v(x,t), t=0,0.4,...,2",xlim=c(xl,xu),
               lty=1,main="v(x,t); t=0,0.4,...,2;",
                  lwd=2);
```

```
    par(mfrow=c(1,1));
    matplot(x=xg,y=s_xplot,type="l",xlab="x",
            ylab="s(x,t), t=0,0.4,...,2",xlim=c(xl,xu),
               lty=1,main="s(x,t); t=0,0.4,...,2;",
                  lwd=2);
  }
```

- For ip=2, three plots for $u(x,t), v(x,t), \sigma(x,t)$ are again produced with matplot. Note the use of the grid in t, vector tout, as the x (horizontal) variable. One dimensional arrays are defined with rep and used as the y (vertical) variable. Point 13 is used corresponding to $x = 0$.

```
#
# vs t at x = 0, t = 0,0.05,...,2
  if(ip==2){
    u_tplot=rep(0,nout);v_tplot=rep(0,nout);
    s_tplot=rep(0,nout);
    for(it in 1:nout){
      u_tplot[it]=u_xplot[13,it];
      v_tplot[it]=v_xplot[13,it];
      s_tplot[it]=s_xplot[13,it];
     }
    par(mfrow=c(1,1));
    matplot(x=tout,y=u_tplot,type="l",xlab="t",
            ylab="u(x,t), x = 0",xlim=c(t0,tf),lty=1,
            main="u(x,t); x = 0",lwd=2);
    par(mfrow=c(1,1));
    matplot(x=tout,y=v_tplot,type="l",xlab="t",
            ylab="v(x,t), x = 0",xlim=c(t0,tf),lty=1,
            main="v(x,t); x = 0",lwd=2);
    par(mfrow=c(1,1));
    matplot(x=tout,y=s_tplot,type="l",xlab="t",
            ylab="s(x,t), x = 0",xlim=c(t0,tf),lty=1,
            main="s(x,t); x = 0",lwd=2);
  }
```

This completes the programming of eqs. (7.1)–(7.3). The computed solutions are considered next.

7.3 Model Output

The parameters defined in the main program of Listing 7.2 are considered to be a base case. Then variations in these parameters are considered, especially `E` in eqs. (7.1a) and (7.1c).

7.3.1 Base Case

The base case parameters are (from Listing 7.2)

```
#
# Parameters
  alpha=0.2; beta=1; gamma=1; D=0.6; E=0.2; kr=1;
  ub=1;      vb=1;   ua=0;
```

The abbreviated output is given in Table 7.1. We can note the following details about this output.

- The solution array `out` from ODE integrator `ode` (with default `lsoda`) has the dimensions 6×79. The row dimension reflects the six values of t. The column dimension reflects the three PDEs (eqs. (7.1)) as $(3)(26) + 1 = 79$. The additional `1` results from the return of values of t as well as the 26 ODE solutions for each of the three PDEs.
- The ICs for $u(x,t=0), v(x,t=0), \sigma(x,t=0)$ (set in Listing 7.3) are verified.
- The output is for $t = 0, 2$ as expected. For $t = 2$, the variation of the solutions with x can be compared with the graphical output to follow.
- The solutions are symmetric with respect to $x = 0$, as expected (there is no preferred direction in x from eqs. (7.1)).
- The computational effort is modest with `ncall` $= 952$.

The plotted solutions are given in Figs. 7.1–7.3 (for $u(x,t)$, $v(x,t), \sigma(x,t)$, respectively). In Fig. 7.1, the solution starts at $u(x,t) = 0.75$ and from top to bottom reaches the solution at $t = 2$ reflected in Table 7.1. This reduction in $u(x,t)$ reflects the departure

TABLE 7.1 Abbreviated output for $u(x,t), v(x,t), \sigma(x,t)$ of eqs. (7.1), ncase=1.

```
 D =   0.600   E =   0.200

 nrow(out)
 [1] 6
 ncol(out)
 [1] 79

      t       x       u(x,t)      v(x,t)      s(x,t)
    0.0   -0.50     0.75000     0.25000     0.00000
    0.0   -0.46     0.75000     0.25000     0.00000
    0.0   -0.42     0.75000     0.25000     0.00000
    0.0   -0.38     0.75000     0.25000     0.00000
    0.0   -0.34     0.75000     0.25000     0.00000
    0.0   -0.30     0.75000     0.25000     0.00000
              .                                .
              .                                .
              .                                .
           Output for x = -0.26 to 0.26 removed
              .                                .
              .                                .
              .                                .
    0.0    0.30     0.75000     0.25000     0.00000
    0.0    0.34     0.75000     0.25000     0.00000
    0.0    0.38     0.75000     0.25000     0.00000
    0.0    0.42     0.75000     0.25000     0.00000
    0.0    0.46     0.75000     0.25000     0.00000
    0.0    0.50     0.75000     0.25000     0.00000

      t       x       u(x,t)      v(x,t)      s(x,t)
    2.0   -0.50     0.05633     0.15719    -0.13054
    2.0   -0.46     0.06032     0.16243    -0.13167
    2.0   -0.42     0.06399     0.16707    -0.13270
    2.0   -0.38     0.06733     0.17116    -0.13363
    2.0   -0.34     0.07035     0.17473    -0.13446
    2.0   -0.30     0.07303     0.17781    -0.13520
              .                                .
```

(continued)

TABLE 7.1 ***(Continued)***

```
         .                                       .
         .                                       .
        Output for x = -0.26 to 0.26 removed
         .                                       .
         .                                       .
         .                                       .
  2.0   0.30      0.07303      0.17781     -0.13520
  2.0   0.34      0.07035      0.17473     -0.13446
  2.0   0.38      0.06733      0.17116     -0.13363
  2.0   0.42      0.06399      0.16707     -0.13270
  2.0   0.46      0.06032      0.16243     -0.13167
  2.0   0.50      0.05633      0.15719     -0.13054

  ncall =    952
```

of the unbound drug from the polymer to the surroundings (at concentration `ua` $= 0$ and the binding/unbinding dynamics.

In Fig. 7.2, the solution starts at $u(x, t = 0) = 0.25$ and goes through a transient to reach the solution at $t = 2$ reflected in

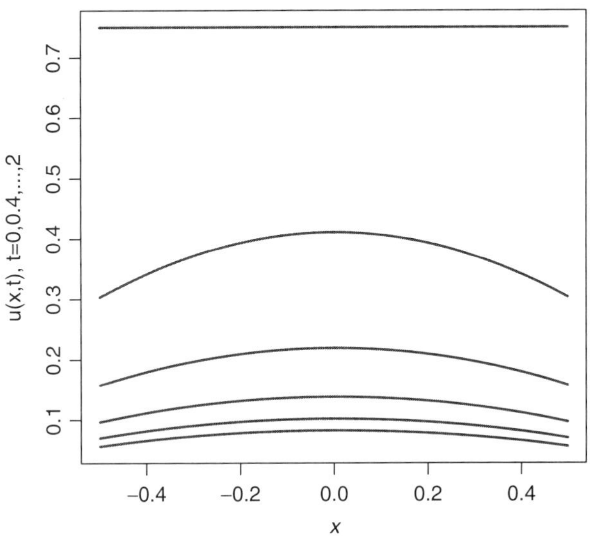

Figure 7.1 $u(x,t)$ versus x, $t = 0, 0.4, \ldots, 2$.

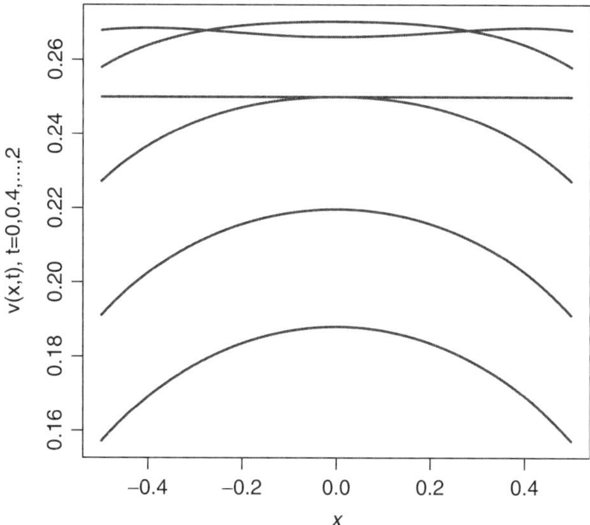

Figure 7.2 $v(x,t)$ versus x, $t = 0, 0.4, \ldots, 2$.

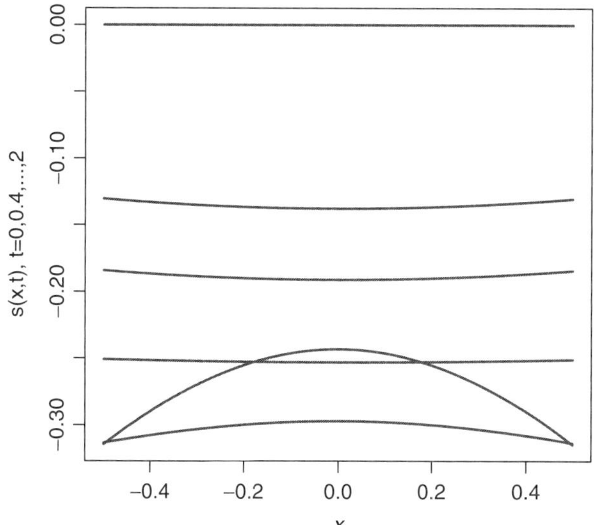

Figure 7.3 $\sigma(x,t)$ vs x, $t = 0, 0.4, \ldots, 2$.

Table 7.1. This reduction in $v(x,t)$ reflects the departure of the bound drug from the polymer to the surroundings by first unbinding.

In Fig. 7.3, the solution starts at $\sigma(x, t = 0) = 0$ and goes through a transient to reach the solution at $t = 2$ reflected in Table 7.1.

This decrease in $\sigma(x,t)$ (to increasingly negative values) reflects the buildup of the stress from an initial zero value as the drug concentrations change. This also suggests that the initial stress set in Listing 7.2 may not be zero.

As the direction of the solution through $t = 0.4, 0.8, \ldots, 2$ requires careful interpretation, especially for Figs. 7.2 and 7.3, an alternative is to label the solution curves and possibly couple the curves to a legend. A variety of graphical formats for this purpose is discussed in [3]. Subsequently, we consider one basic format for labeling the curves.

For `ip=2` in Listing 7.3, the three plots of the solution at $x = 0$ as a function of t are given in Figs. 7.4–7.6.

Fig. 7.4 indicates that $u(x = 0, t)$ approaches a steady state at $t = 2$ that could eventually (with large t) be close to zero as the unbound drug exits the polymer (at the boundaries $x = -x_l, x_l$).

Fig. 7.5 indicates that $v(x = 0, t)$ lags the response of $u(x = 0, t)$ in Fig. 7.4 but steadily declines as the bound drug is unbound and then exits the polymer.

Fig. 7.6 indicates that the stress $\sigma(x,t)$ approaches a negative value at $t = 2$ that suggests a residual compression as the drug exits the

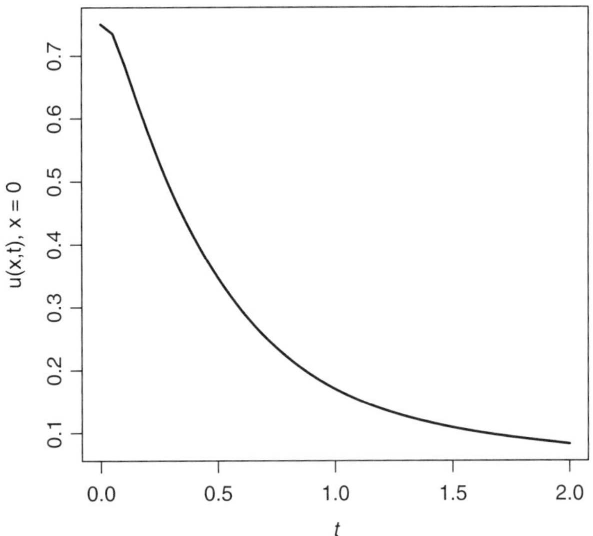

Figure 7.4 $u(x,t)$ versus t, $x = 0$.

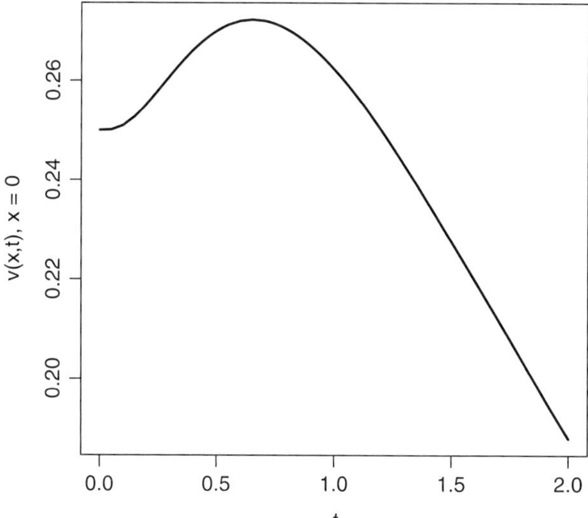

Figure 7.5 $v(x,t)$ versus t, $x = 0$.

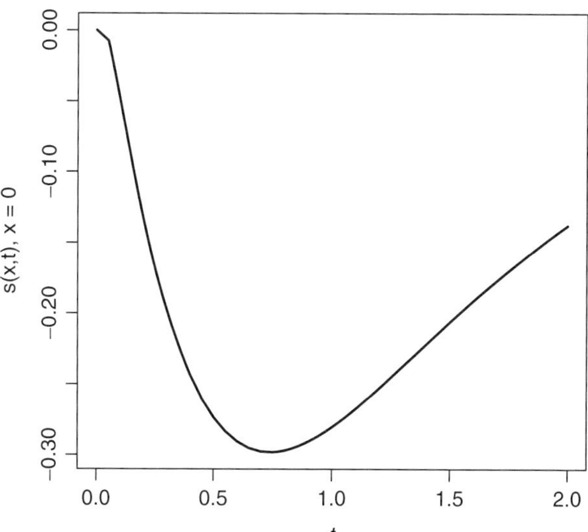

Figure 7.6 $\sigma(x,t)$ versus t, $x = 0$.

polymer. This $\sigma(x = 0, t = 2)$ value is consistent with the value of $\sigma(x, t = 2)$ in Table 7.1.

Finally, to elucidate the evolution of the solutions in t in Figs. 7.1–7.3, the individual solutions are plotted with identifying numbers through Listing 7.4 (used in Listing 7.3 in place of the previous code for $u(x, t), v(x, t), \sigma(x, t)$ vs x).

```
#
# Plot u,v,s numerical solutions
#
# vs x with t as a parameter, t = 0,0.4,...,2
  if(ip==1){
#
#   t=0
    par(mfrow=c(1,1));
    plot(xg,u_xplot[,1],type="b",lty=1,pch="1",xlab="x",
    ylab="u(x,t),t=0,0.4,...,2",xlim=c(xl,xu),ylim=
       c(0,0.8),main="u(x,t); t=0,0.4,...,2;",lwd=2)
#
#   t=0.4,0.8,1.2,1.6,2
    lines(xg,u_xplot[,2],type="b",lty=1,pch="2",lwd=2)
    lines(xg,u_xplot[,3],type="b",lty=1,pch="3",lwd=2)
    lines(xg,u_xplot[,4],type="b",lty=1,pch="4",lwd=2)
    lines(xg,u_xplot[,5],type="b",lty=1,pch="5",lwd=2)
    lines(xg,u_xplot[,6],type="b",lty=1,pch="6",lwd=2)
#
#   t=0
    par(mfrow=c(1,1));
    plot(xg,v_xplot[,1],type="b",lty=1,pch="1",xlab="x",
    ylab="v(x,t),t=0,0.4,...,2",xlim=c(xl,xu),ylim=
       c(0.1,0.3),main="v(x,t); t=0,0.4,...,2;",lwd=2)
#
#   t=0.4,0.8,1.2,1.6,2
    lines(xg,v_xplot[,2],type="b",lty=1,pch="2",lwd=2)
    lines(xg,v_xplot[,3],type="b",lty=1,pch="3",lwd=2)
    lines(xg,v_xplot[,4],type="b",lty=1,pch="4",lwd=2)
    lines(xg,v_xplot[,5],type="b",lty=1,pch="5",lwd=2)
    lines(xg,v_xplot[,6],type="b",lty=1,pch="6",lwd=2)
#
#   t=0
    par(mfrow=c(1,1));
```

```
    plot(xg,s_xplot[,1],type="b",lty=1,pch="1",xlab="x",
    ylab="s(x,t),t=0,0.4,...,2",xlim=c(xl,xu),ylim=
       c(-0.4,0.0),main="s(x,t); t=0,0.4,...,2;",lwd=2)
#
#   t=0.4,0.8,1.2,1.6,2
    lines(xg,s_xplot[,2],type="b",lty=1,pch="2",lwd=2)
    lines(xg,s_xplot[,3],type="b",lty=1,pch="3",lwd=2)
    lines(xg,s_xplot[,4],type="b",lty=1,pch="4",lwd=2)
    lines(xg,s_xplot[,5],type="b",lty=1,pch="5",lwd=2)
    lines(xg,s_xplot[,6],type="b",lty=1,pch="6",lwd=2)
  }
```

Listing 7.4 Modification of plotting to identify solutions with numbered points.

The output from Listing 7.4 is in Figs. 7.7–7.9. We can note the following details about this code.

- `matplot` of Listing 7.3 is replaced with `plot`.
- `lines` is used to produce the solution at $t = 0.4$ (from `u_xplot[,2]`) to $t = 2$ (from `u_xplot[,6]`). The argument

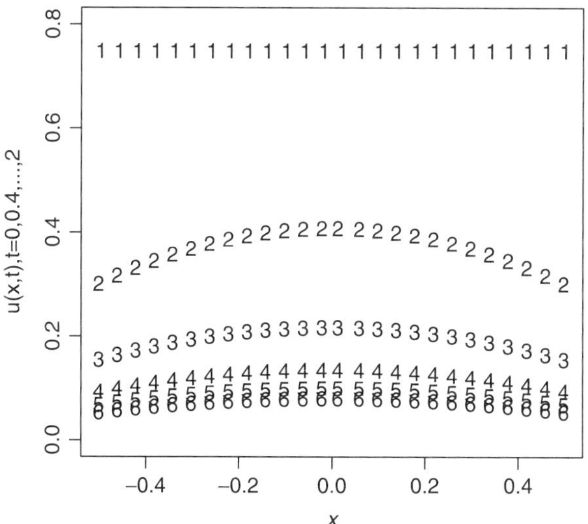

Figure 7.7 $u(x,t)$ versus x, $t = 0, 0.4, \ldots, 2$ from Listing 7.4.

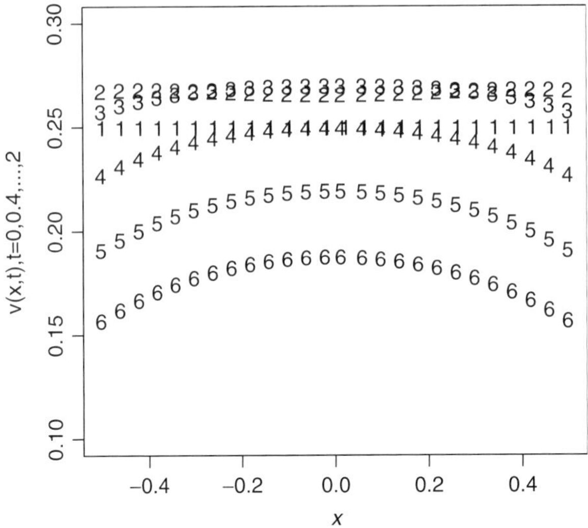

Figure 7.8 $v(x,t)$ versus x, $t = 0, 0.4, \ldots, 2$ from Listing 7.4.

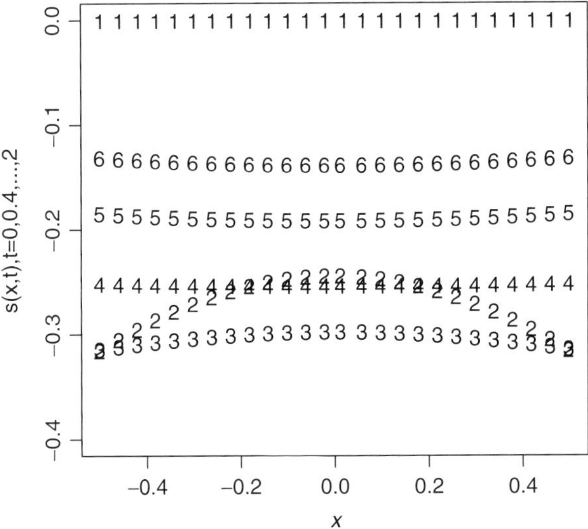

Figure 7.9 $\sigma(x,t)$ versus x, $t = 0, 0.4, \ldots, 2$ from Listing 7.4.

`[,2]`, for example, specifies all values of x at $t = 0.4$ so $u(x,t = 0.4)$ is plotted against x (in `xg`).

- In each call to `lines`, the parameter `pch` is used to specify a numerical character for each point in the plot (see Figs. 7.7–7.9).

- `ylim=c(0,0.8)` in the first call to `plot` specifies a range in the vertical axis of $0 \leq u(x,t) \leq 0.8$. This range covers all values of $u(x,t)$ in the subsequent five calls to `lines`. This is an important detail because if $u(x,t)$ in the calls to `lines` goes outside this range, `lines` is not executed. Note also `ylim=c(0.1,0.3)` for $v(x,t)$ and `ylim=c(-0.4,0.0)` for $\sigma(x,t)$, which are consistent with the vertical variation in $v(x,t)$ and $\sigma(x,t)$ in Figs. 7.2 and 7.3, and Figs. 7.8 and 7.9.

In summary, this use of `plot` and `lines` elucidates the variation of the solutions with t in Figs. 7.1–7.3 by comparison with Figs. 7.7–7.9.

7.3.2 Variation of Spatial Differentiation

`drug_1` in Listing 7.1 is based on the use of stagewise differentiation (two successive calls to `dss004` to give the second derivatives in x in eqs. (7.1a) and (7.1c)). An alternative is to calculate the second derivatives directly as programmed in ODE routine `drug_2` in Listing 7.5 next.

```
  drug_2=function(t,U,parms){
#
# Function drug_2 computes the t derivative vector
# of the u,v,s vectors
#
# One vector to three vectors
  u=rep(0,nx);v=rep(0,nx);
  s=rep(0,nx);
  for(i in 1:nx){
    u[i]=U[i];
    v[i]=U[i+nx];
    s[i]=U[i+2*nx];
  }
#
# ux, sx
# ux=dss004(xl,xu,nx,u);
# sx=dss004(xl,xu,nx,s);
#
```

```
# Boundary conditions
  ux=rep(0,nx);sx=rep(0,nx);
  ux[1]=-(kr/D)*(ua-u[1]);
  ux[nx]=(kr/D)*(ua-u[nx]);
  sx[1]=0;sx[nx]=0;
#
# uxx, sxx
  nl=2;nu=2;
  uxx=dss044(xl,xu,nx,u,ux,nl,nu);
  sxx=dss044(xl,xu,nx,s,sx,nl,nu);
#
# PDEs
  ut=rep(0,nx);vt=rep(0,nx)
  st=rep(0,nx);
  for(i in 1:nx){
    ut[i]=D*uxx[i]+E*sxx[i]+f_u(ub,vb,u[i],v[i]);
    vt[i]=g_v(ub,vb,u[i],v[i]);
    st[i]=alpha*u[i]-beta*s[i]+gamma*ut[i];
  }
#
# Three vectors to one vector
  Ut=rep(0,3*nx);
  for(i in 1:nx){
    Ut[i]     =ut[i];
    Ut[i+nx]  =vt[i];
    Ut[i+2*nx]=st[i];
  }
#
# Increment calls to drug_2
  ncall <<- ncall+1;
#
# Return derivative vector
  return(list(c(Ut)));
}
```

Listing 7.5 ODE routine drug_2 for eqs. (7.1) and (7.3).

drug_2 is called by ode in the main program of Listing 7.3 with ncase=2, whereas drug_1 is called with ncase1=1.

```
#
# ODE integration
```

```
if(ncase==1){
  out=ode(y=u0,times=tout,func=drug_1,parms=NULL);}
if(ncase==2){
  out=ode(y=u0,times=tout,func=drug_2,parms=NULL);}
```

We can note the following details about drug_2 of Listing 7.5 (with emphasis on the differences from drug_1 of Listing 7.1).

- The function drug_2 is defined and the three 1D vectors u,v,s are utilized as in Listing 7.1 for u, v, s of eqs. (7.1).
- dss004 is not used to compute the first derivatives in x as in Listing 7.1 (the calls are deactivated as comments). Rather, the vectors ux,vx,sx are defined with a rep.

```
#
# ux, sx
# ux=dss004(xl,xu,nx,u);
# sx=dss004(xl,xu,nx,s);
#
# Boundary conditions
  ux=rep(0,nx);sx=rep(0,nx);
  ux[1]=-(kr/D)*(ua-u[1]);
  ux[nx]=(kr/D)*(ua-u[nx]);
  sx[1]=0;sx[nx]=0;
```

  The derivatives $\partial u(x = -x_l, t)/\partial x, \partial u(x = x_l, t)/\partial x$ of eqs. (7.3e,f) are programmed (as ux[1],ux[nx]). Then the derivatives $\partial \sigma(x = -x_l, t)/\partial x, \partial \sigma(x = x_l, t)/\partial x$ of eqs. (7.3i,j) are programmed (as sx[1],sx[nx]).
- The second derivatives $\partial^2 u(x,t)/\partial x^2$,$\partial^2 \sigma(x,t)/\partial x^2$ of eqs. (7.1a) and (7.1c) are computed by dss044.

```
#
# uxx, sxx
  nl=2;nu=2;
  uxx=dss044(xl,xu,nx,u,ux,nl,nu);
  sxx=dss044(xl,xu,nx,s,sx,nl,nu);
```

Neumann BCs are specified with `nl=nu=2`. Also, only the boundary values of the first derivatives, `ux[1],ux[nx], sx[1],sx[nx]`, are used by `dss044` (interior values of the first derivatives in x are not required by `dss044`).

- Eqs. (7.1) are programmed as in Listing 7.1. Also, the derivatives in t (`Ut`) are returned to `ode` as in Listing 7.1.

The abbreviated numerical output from `drug_2` (called by the main program of Listing 7.3 with `ncase=2`) is given in Table 7.2.

We can note the following details about this output.

- The numerical values of Tables 7.1 and 7.2 are nearly the same. For example,

```
Table 7.1 (ncase=1)

    t       x         u(x,t)        v(x,t)        s(x,t)
   2.0   -0.50       0.05633       0.15719      -0.13054
   2.0   -0.46       0.06032       0.16243      -0.13167
   2.0   -0.42       0.06399       0.16707      -0.13270
   2.0   -0.38       0.06733       0.17116      -0.13363
   2.0   -0.34       0.07035       0.17473      -0.13446
   2.0   -0.30       0.07303       0.17781      -0.13520

Table 7.2 (ncase=2)

    t       x         u(x,t)        v(x,t)        s(x,t)
   2.0   -0.50       0.05633       0.15719      -0.13054
   2.0   -0.46       0.06032       0.16243      -0.13167
   2.0   -0.42       0.06399       0.16707      -0.13270
   2.0   -0.38       0.06733       0.17116      -0.13363
   2.0   -0.34       0.07035       0.17473      -0.13446
   2.0   -0.30       0.07303       0.17782      -0.13520
```

- `drug_2` was called somewhat more than `drug_1`.

```
drug_1: ncall = 952

drug_2: ncall = 1223
```

TABLE 7.2 Abbreviated output for $u(x,t), v(x,t), \sigma(x,t)$ of eqs. (7.1), ncase=2.

```
D =  0.600   E =  0.200

nrow(out)
[1] 6
ncol(out)
[1] 79

   t       x       u(x,t)       v(x,t)       s(x,t)
  0.0   -0.50     0.75000      0.25000      0.00000
  0.0   -0.46     0.75000      0.25000      0.00000
  0.0   -0.42     0.75000      0.25000      0.00000
  0.0   -0.38     0.75000      0.25000      0.00000
  0.0   -0.34     0.75000      0.25000      0.00000
  0.0   -0.30     0.75000      0.25000      0.00000
          .                                    .
          .                                    .
          .                                    .
        Output for x = -0.26 to 0.26 removed
          .                                    .
          .                                    .
          .                                    .
  0.0    0.30     0.75000      0.25000      0.00000
  0.0    0.34     0.75000      0.25000      0.00000
  0.0    0.38     0.75000      0.25000      0.00000
  0.0    0.42     0.75000      0.25000      0.00000
  0.0    0.46     0.75000      0.25000      0.00000
  0.0    0.50     0.75000      0.25000      0.00000

   t       x       u(x,t)       v(x,t)       s(x,t)
  2.0   -0.50     0.05633      0.15719     -0.13054
  2.0   -0.46     0.06032      0.16243     -0.13167
  2.0   -0.42     0.06399      0.16707     -0.13270
  2.0   -0.38     0.06733      0.17116     -0.13363
  2.0   -0.34     0.07035      0.17473     -0.13446
  2.0   -0.30     0.07303      0.17782     -0.13520
          .                                    .
```

(continued)

TABLE 7.2 (*Continued*)

```
             .                                .
             .                                .
          Output for x = -0.26 to 0.26 removed
             .                                .
             .                                .
             .                                .
     2.0    0.30       0.07303      0.17782    -0.13520
     2.0    0.34       0.07035      0.17473    -0.13446
     2.0    0.38       0.06733      0.17116    -0.13363
     2.0    0.42       0.06399      0.16707    -0.13270
     2.0    0.46       0.06032      0.16243    -0.13167
     2.0    0.50       0.05633      0.15719    -0.13054

     ncall =   1223
```

In summary, for eqs. (7.1), stagewise differentiation and direct differentiation produced essentially the same results. The intent here is to demonstrate the alternative MOL calculations.

7.3.3 Variation of Polymer Stress

With an operational code for eqs. (7.1)–(7.3), we now briefly consider some of the characteristics of these equations by varying the parameter E in eqs. (7.1a) and (7.1c). For $E = -0.2$ (a sign change in the base case value), the main program of Listing 7.3 gives the abbreviated output listed in Table 7.3.

The output in Table 7.3 is different from that in Table 7.1 (for $E = 0.2$), but the difference is not large as indicated by the following comparison.

```
E=0.2 (Table 7.1)

     t        x        u(x,t)       v(x,t)        s(x,t)
    2.0   -0.50       0.05633      0.15719      -0.13054
    2.0   -0.46       0.06032      0.16243      -0.13167
    2.0   -0.42       0.06399      0.16707      -0.13270
    2.0   -0.38       0.06733      0.17116      -0.13363
```

TABLE 7.3 Abbreviated output for $u(x,t)$, $v(x,t)$, $\sigma(x,t)$ of eqs. (7.1), ncase=1, $E = -0.2$.

```
D =   0.600    E = -0.200

nrow(out)
[1] 6
ncol(out)
[1] 79

    t        x        u(x,t)        v(x,t)        s(x,t)
  0.0    -0.50      0.75000       0.25000       0.00000
  0.0    -0.46      0.75000       0.25000       0.00000
  0.0    -0.42      0.75000       0.25000       0.00000
  0.0    -0.38      0.75000       0.25000       0.00000
  0.0    -0.34      0.75000       0.25000       0.00000
  0.0    -0.30      0.75000       0.25000       0.00000
             .                                  .
             .                                  .
             .                                  .
        Output for x = -0.26 to 0.26 removed
             .                                  .
             .                                  .
             .                                  .
  0.0     0.30      0.75000       0.25000       0.00000
  0.0     0.34      0.75000       0.25000       0.00000
  0.0     0.38      0.75000       0.25000       0.00000
  0.0     0.42      0.75000       0.25000       0.00000
  0.0     0.46      0.75000       0.25000       0.00000
  0.0     0.50      0.75000       0.25000       0.00000

    t        x        u(x,t)        v(x,t)        s(x,t)
  2.0    -0.50      0.06024       0.16287      -0.12954
  2.0    -0.46      0.06316       0.16836      -0.13239
  2.0    -0.42      0.06584       0.17311      -0.13502
  2.0    -0.38      0.06828       0.17717      -0.13743
  2.0    -0.34      0.07049       0.18062      -0.13962
  2.0    -0.30      0.07245       0.18351      -0.14157
             .                                  .
             .                                  .
```

(continued)

TABLE 7.3 *(Continued)*

```
                .                                      .
                Output for x = -0.26 to 0.26 removed
                .                                      .
                .                                      .
                .                                      .
   2.0   0.30      0.07245      0.18351     -0.14157
   2.0   0.34      0.07049      0.18062     -0.13962
   2.0   0.38      0.06828      0.17717     -0.13743
   2.0   0.42      0.06584      0.17311     -0.13502
   2.0   0.46      0.06316      0.16836     -0.13239
   2.0   0.50      0.06024      0.16287     -0.12954

   ncall =    850
```

```
2.0   -0.34     0.07035     0.17473     -0.13446
2.0   -0.30     0.07303     0.17781     -0.13520
```

```
E=-0.2 (Table 7.3)

   t      x        u(x,t)       v(x,t)       s(x,t)
 2.0   -0.50     0.06024      0.16287      -0.12954
 2.0   -0.46     0.06316      0.16836      -0.13239
 2.0   -0.42     0.06584      0.17311      -0.13502
 2.0   -0.38     0.06828      0.17717      -0.13743
 2.0   -0.34     0.07049      0.18062      -0.13962
 2.0   -0.30     0.07245      0.18351      -0.14157
```

Thus, changing from $E = 0.2$ to $E = -0.2$ did not produce a large effect (i.e., E is not a sensitive parameter in the range -0.2 to 0.2). This conclusion is confirmed by comparing Fig. 7.10 (for $v(x, t)$ with $E = -0.2$) with Fig. 7.2, which shows a relatively small vertical shifting of the solution curves.

For $E = 2$, the main program of Listing 7.3 gives the abbreviated output listed in Table 7.4.

The output in Table 7.4 is different from that in Table 7.1 (for $E = 0.2$), but again, the difference is not qualitatively different as indicated by the following comparison.

TABLE 7.4 Abbreviated output for $u(x,t), v(x,t), \sigma(x,t)$ of eqs. (7.1), ncase=1, $E = 2$.

```
 D =   0.600    E =   2.000

 nrow(out)
 [1] 6
 ncol(out)
 [1] 79

     t       x       u(x,t)       v(x,t)       s(x,t)
   0.0   -0.50     0.75000      0.25000      0.00000
   0.0   -0.46     0.75000      0.25000      0.00000
   0.0   -0.42     0.75000      0.25000      0.00000
   0.0   -0.38     0.75000      0.25000      0.00000
   0.0   -0.34     0.75000      0.25000      0.00000
   0.0   -0.30     0.75000      0.25000      0.00000
             .                                 .
             .                                 .
             .                                 .
         Output for x = -0.26 to 0.26 removed
             .                                 .
             .                                 .
             .                                 .
   0.0    0.30     0.75000      0.25000      0.00000
   0.0    0.34     0.75000      0.25000      0.00000
   0.0    0.38     0.75000      0.25000      0.00000
   0.0    0.42     0.75000      0.25000      0.00000
   0.0    0.46     0.75000      0.25000      0.00000
   0.0    0.50     0.75000      0.25000      0.00000

     t       x       u(x,t)       v(x,t)       s(x,t)
   2.0   -0.50     0.05303      0.15404     -0.13339
   2.0   -0.46     0.05586      0.15689     -0.13323
   2.0   -0.42     0.05845      0.15946     -0.13307
   2.0   -0.38     0.06081      0.16178     -0.13293
   2.0   -0.34     0.06292      0.16384     -0.13280
   2.0   -0.30     0.06480      0.16565     -0.13268
             .                                 .
             .                                 .
```

(continued)

TABLE 7.4 (*Continued*)

```
          .                                  .
          Output for x = -0.26 to 0.26 removed
          .                                  .
          .                                  .
          .                                  .
    2.0   0.30      0.06480      0.16565     -0.13268
    2.0   0.34      0.06292      0.16384     -0.13280
    2.0   0.38      0.06081      0.16178     -0.13293
    2.0   0.42      0.05845      0.15946     -0.13307
    2.0   0.46      0.05586      0.15689     -0.13323
    2.0   0.50      0.05303      0.15404     -0.13339

    ncall =   1083
```

```
E=0.2 (Table 7.1)

    t       x      u(x,t)      v(x,t)      s(x,t)
  2.0   -0.50     0.05633     0.15719    -0.13054
  2.0   -0.46     0.06032     0.16243    -0.13167
  2.0   -0.42     0.06399     0.16707    -0.13270
  2.0   -0.38     0.06733     0.17116    -0.13363
```

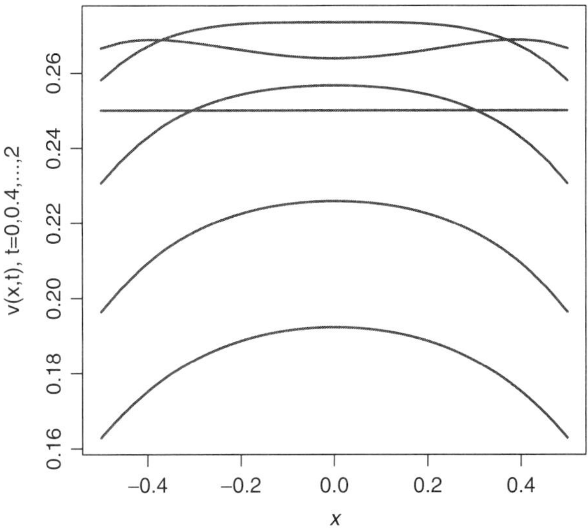

Figure 7.10 $v(x,t)$ versus x, $t = 0, 0.4, \ldots, 2$, $E = -0.2$.

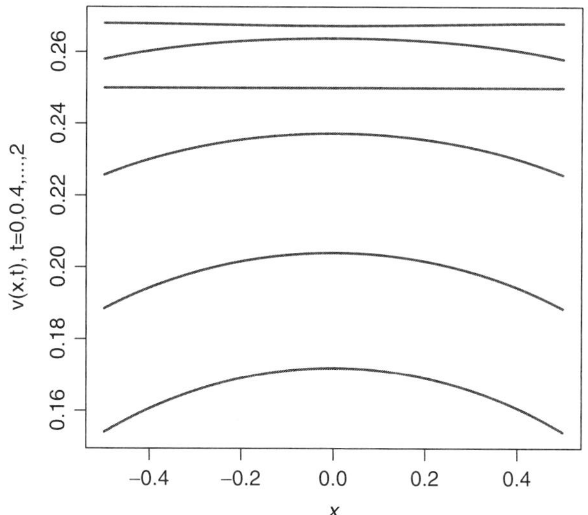

Figure 7.11 $v(x,t)$ versus x, $t = 0, 0.4, \ldots, 2$, $E = 2$.

```
   2.0   -0.34       0.07035       0.17473       -0.13446
   2.0   -0.30       0.07303       0.17781       -0.13520

E=2 (Table 7.4)
     t        x        u(x,t)        v(x,t)          s(x,t)
   2.0   -0.50       0.05303       0.15404       -0.13339
   2.0   -0.46       0.05586       0.15689       -0.13323
   2.0   -0.42       0.05845       0.15946       -0.13307
   2.0   -0.38       0.06081       0.16178       -0.13293
   2.0   -0.34       0.06292       0.16384       -0.13280
   2.0   -0.30       0.06480       0.16565       -0.13268
```

Thus, changing from $E = 0.2$ to $E = 2$ did not produce a large effect (i.e., E is not a sensitive parameter in the range 0.2 to 2). This conclusion is confirmed by comparing Fig. 7.11 (for $v(x,t)$ with $E = 2$) with Fig. 7.2, which shows a relatively small vertical shifting of the solution curves.

7.4 Alternate Coordinate Systems

Eqs. (7.1a,c) are stated in Cartesian coordinates through the spatial variable x. Furthermore, eqs. (7.1a,c) are 1D as a special case of a

3D coordinate system (x, y, z). Such a 1D "slab" may not represent the physical system of interest very well (this special case was used to follow the original reference [1]). Other coordinate systems can be considered that better conform to the physical shape of the problem system. Two other coordinates frequently used in PDE models are (1) cylindrical with coordinates (r, θ, z) and (2) spherical with coordinates (r, θ, ϕ). To illustrate how PDEs in these two coordinate system originate, we consider a derivation in 1D for the radial coordinate only (a derivation of the 3D diffusion equation in cylindrical and spherical coordinates is given in [2], Appendix 1).

For cylindrical coordinates, a mass balance on an incremental volume $2\pi r z_l dr$ (where z_l is the length in z and variations in the angle θ and axial coordinate z are neglected) gives

$$\begin{aligned}2\pi r z_l dr\frac{\partial u}{\partial t} &= 2\pi(r+dr)z_l D\left.\frac{\partial u}{\partial r}\right|_{r+dr} - 2\pi r z_l D\left.\frac{\partial u}{\partial r}\right|_{r} \\ &\quad + 2\pi(r+dr)z_l E\left.\frac{\partial \sigma}{\partial r}\right|_{r+dr} - 2\pi r z_l E\left.\frac{\partial \sigma}{\partial r}\right|_{r} \\ &\quad + 2\pi r z_l dr f(u, v)\end{aligned} \tag{7.4a}$$

where we have made use of Fick's first law for the diffusive flux q_r in the r-direction, for example,

$$q_r = -D\frac{\partial u}{\partial r} \tag{7.4b}$$

The second line in eq. (7.4a) accounts for a radial diffusion flux resulting from the radial variation of the stress in the polymer. The third line indicates that $f(u, v)$ is a volumetric source function (it is multiplied by the incremental volume $2\pi r z_l dr$).

Division of eq. (7.4a) by the incremental volume $2\pi r z_l dr$ gives

$$\begin{aligned}\frac{\partial u}{\partial t} &= \frac{(r+dr)D\left.\dfrac{\partial u}{\partial r}\right|_{r+dr} - rD\left.\dfrac{\partial u}{\partial r}\right|_{r}}{rdr} \\ &\quad + \frac{(r+dr)E\left.\dfrac{\partial \sigma}{\partial r}\right|_{r+dr} - rE\left.\dfrac{\partial \sigma}{\partial r}\right|_{r}}{rdr} + f(u, v)\end{aligned} \tag{7.4c}$$

In the limit $dr \to 0$, eq. (7.4c) becomes

$$\frac{\partial u}{\partial t} = \frac{1}{r}\frac{\partial}{\partial r}\left[rD\frac{\partial u}{\partial r}\right] + \frac{1}{r}\frac{\partial}{\partial r}\left[rE\frac{\partial \sigma}{\partial r}\right] + f(u,v) \tag{7.4d}$$

or for constant D, E,

$$\frac{\partial u}{\partial t} = D\left[\frac{\partial^2 u}{\partial r^2} + \frac{1}{r}\frac{\partial u}{\partial r}\right] + E\left[\frac{\partial^2 \sigma}{\partial r^2} + \frac{1}{r}\frac{\partial \sigma}{\partial r}\right] + f(u,v) \tag{7.4e}$$

Eq. (7.4e) is the equivalent of eq. (7.1a) in cylindrical coordinates.

For spherical coordinates, the derivation is very similar. A mass balance on an incremental volume $4\pi r^2 dr$ gives (where variations in the angles θ and ϕ are neglected)

$$\begin{aligned} 4\pi r^2 dr\frac{\partial u}{\partial t} &= 4\pi(r+dr)^2 D\left.\frac{\partial u}{\partial r}\right|_{r+dr} - 4\pi r^2 D\left.\frac{\partial u}{\partial r}\right|_{r} \\ &\quad + 4\pi(r+dr)^2 E\left.\frac{\partial \sigma}{\partial r}\right|_{r+dr} - 4\pi r^2 E\left.\frac{\partial \sigma}{\partial r}\right|_{r} \\ &\quad + 4\pi r^2 dr\, f(u,v) \end{aligned} \tag{7.5a}$$

where we have again made use of Fick's first law for the diffusive flux q_r in the r-direction, for example,

$$q_r = -D\frac{\partial u}{\partial r} \tag{7.5b}$$

Division of eq. (7.5a) by the incremental volume $4\pi r^2 dr$ gives

$$\begin{aligned} \frac{\partial u}{\partial t} &= \frac{(r+dr)^2 D\left.\frac{\partial u}{\partial r}\right|_{r+dr} - r^2 D\left.\frac{\partial u}{\partial r}\right|_{r}}{r^2 dr} \\ &\quad + \frac{(r+dr)^2 E\left.\frac{\partial \sigma}{\partial r}\right|_{r+dr} - r^2 E\left.\frac{\partial \sigma}{\partial r}\right|_{r}}{r^2 dr} + f(u,v) \end{aligned} \tag{7.5c}$$

In the limit $dr \to 0$, eq. (7.5c) becomes

$$\frac{\partial u}{\partial t} = \frac{1}{r^2}\frac{\partial}{\partial r}\left[r^2 D\frac{\partial u}{\partial r}\right] + \frac{1}{r^2}\frac{\partial}{\partial r}\left[r^2 E\frac{\partial \sigma}{\partial r}\right] + f(u,v) \tag{7.5d}$$

or for constant D, E,

$$\frac{\partial u}{\partial t} = D\left[\frac{\partial^2 u}{\partial r^2} + \frac{2}{r}\frac{\partial u}{\partial r}\right] + E\left[\frac{\partial^2 \sigma}{\partial r^2} + \frac{2}{r}\frac{\partial \sigma}{\partial r}\right] + f(u, v) \qquad (7.5e)$$

Eq. (7.5e) is the equivalent of eq. (7.1a) in spherical coordinates.

The MOL solution of eqs. (7.4e) and (7.5e) is very similar to the preceding solution for eq. (7.1a). One additional difference pertains to the range or interval in r. While the interval in x for eqs. (7.1a) and (7.1c) is $-x_l \le x \le x_l$, for r, it is $0 \le r \le r_0$ where r_0 is the outer radius in cylindrical or spherical coordinates. At $r = 0$, a symmetry BC is used, $\partial u(r = 0, t)/\partial r = 0$.

This idea of a symmetry BC could also be used for eqs. (7.1a) and (7.1c) with $0 \le x \le x_l$. In fact, the solutions in Tables 7.1–7.4 demonstrate the symmetry of the solutions around $x = 0$. This suggests that only the half interval $0 \le x \le x_l$ is required for the solutions of eqs. (7.1)–(7.3), which would be worth using because only half of the grid points in x are required. In general, employing symmetries can lead to a reduction in the number of ODEs, and therefore, the effort to compute a numerical solution.

MOL solutions in cylindrical and spherical coordinates are discussed in [2]. Also, solutions in 2D and 3D are discussed in this reference.

7.5 Summary

In conclusion, the effect of polymer stress $\sigma(x, t)$ through the term $E\partial^2\sigma/\partial x^2$ appears qualitatively to be minor for the range of values of E that was studied, $-0.2 \le E \le 2$. The question then arises of why E has a relatively small effect. This question could be studied and probably answered by computing and comparing the various RHS terms in eqs. (7.1a) and (7.1c). For example, $D\partial^2 u/\partial x^2$ and $E\partial^2\sigma/\partial x^2$ are easily computed from the available solutions $u(x, t)$ and $\sigma(x, t)$. We will not go further with this analysis, but conclude by pointing out that the comparison of the various RHS PDE terms, which are available once the numerical solution is computed, gives a direct indication of the contribution of each of the terms and therefore a detailed understanding of the characteristics of the PDE solutions.

References

[1] Ferreira, J.A., P. de Oliveira, and P. da Silva (2012), Analytics and numerics of drug release tracking, *J. Comput. Appl. Math.*, **236**, 3572–3583.

[2] Schiesser, W.E., and G.W. Griffiths (2009), *A Compendium of Partial Differential Equation Models*, Cambridge University Press, Cambridge, UK.

[3] Soetaert, K., J. Cash, and F. Mazzia (2012), *Solving Differential Equations in R*, Springer-Verlag, Heidelberg, Germany.

CHAPTER 8

Temperature Distributions in Cryosurgery

8.1 Introduction

Cryosurgery (surgery at a low temperature) is used to inactivate tumor cells in the treatment of cancer. This form of surgery offers the possibility of an accurately selected (defined) target volume and thus can incur minimum damage to surrounding normal (healthy) tissue. To assess the outcome of a proposed cryosurgical procedure, we consider a mathematical model that provides the distribution of temperatures in the region around the point of treatment.

The domain for cryogenic surgery is illustrated in Fig. 8.1. The cylindrical domain has the dimensions $0 \leq r \leq r_c, 0 \leq z \leq z_c$. A cryoprobe occupies the cylindrical subdomain $0 \leq r \leq r_p, 0 \leq z \leq z_p$. The effect of the probe tip at temperature $T_p(t)$ is of particular interest. In this chapter, we consider the following topics.

- Development of a PDE model for the temperature distribution during cryosurgery. The PDE is 2D in cylindrical coordinates as suggested by Fig. 8.1. Also, it has a variable coefficient that forms a singularity and nonlinear coefficients resulting from temperature-dependent physical properties.

Differential Equation Analysis in Biomedical Science and Engineering: Partial Differential Equation Applications with R, First Edition. William E. Schiesser.

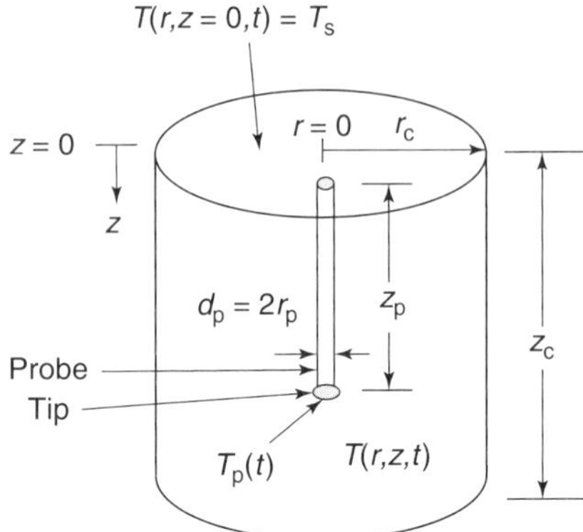

Figure 8.1 Diagrammatic illustration of the region for cryosurgery.

- Algorithms and computer routines for the numerical solution of the model equations.
- Features of the model numerical solutions pertaining to temperature distribution during cryosurgery.
- Graphical output that encompasses three independent variables.

8.2 PDE Model

As indicated in Fig. 8.1, the PDE model will be formulated in cylindrical coordinates, (r, θ, z), starting with the heat conduction equation [1, eq. (A.1.4)].

$$C\frac{\partial T}{\partial t} = \nabla \cdot (\mathbf{k} \cdot \nabla T) \tag{8.1a}$$

where

Variable, Parameter	Interpretation
T	tissue temperature (°C)
t	time (s)
∇	differential operator (1/cm)
C	tissue volumetric heat capacity (J/cm^3 °C)
$\mathbf{k}$	nine-component tissue thermal conductivity tensor (W cm/cm^2 °C)

The RHS of eq. (8.1a) in cylindrical coordinates is ([2], p 390)

$$
\begin{aligned}
\nabla \cdot (\mathbf{k} \cdot \nabla T) = & \frac{1}{r}\frac{\partial}{\partial r}\left(rk_{rr}\frac{\partial T}{\partial r} + rk_{r\theta}\frac{1}{r}\frac{\partial T}{\partial \theta} + rk_{rz}\frac{\partial T}{\partial z}\right) \\
& + \frac{1}{r}\frac{\partial}{\partial \theta}\left(k_{\theta r}\frac{\partial T}{\partial r} + k_{\theta\theta}\frac{1}{r}\frac{\partial T}{\partial \theta} + k_{\theta z}\frac{\partial T}{\partial z}\right) \\
& + \frac{\partial}{\partial z}\left(k_{zr}\frac{\partial T}{\partial r} + k_{z\theta}\frac{1}{r}\frac{\partial T}{\partial \theta} + k_{zz}\frac{\partial T}{\partial z}\right)
\end{aligned} \quad (8.1b)
$$

where

Variable, Parameter	Interpretation
r	radial coordinate (cm)
θ	angular coordinate (radians)
z	axial coordinate (cm)
$k_{rr}, k_{r\theta}, k_{rz}$ $k_{\theta r}, k_{\theta\theta}, k_{\theta z}$ $k_{zr}, k_{z\theta}, k_{zz}$	components of the conductivity tensor in cylindrical coordinates (W m/m^2 °C)

For the case $k_{rr} = k_{\theta\theta} = k_{zz} = k$, $k_{r\theta} = k_{rz} = k_{\theta r} = k_{\theta z} = k_{zr} = k_{z\theta} = 0$ (diagonal terms of the conductivity tensor are equal to k, off-diagonal terms of the conductivity tensor are zero), eq. (8.1b) is

$$
C\frac{\partial T}{\partial t} = \frac{1}{r}\frac{\partial}{\partial r}\left(rk\frac{\partial T}{\partial r}\right) + \frac{1}{r}\frac{\partial}{\partial \theta}\left(k\frac{1}{r}\frac{\partial T}{\partial \theta}\right) + \frac{\partial}{\partial z}\left(k\frac{\partial T}{\partial z}\right) \quad (8.1c)
$$

Eq. (8.1c) is now extended for application to heat conduction in tissue through the inclusion of an additional inhomogeneous term [1]. Also, initially, we assume angular symmetry so that terms in θ are dropped.

$$
C\frac{\partial T}{\partial t} = \frac{1}{r}\frac{\partial}{\partial r}\left(rk\frac{\partial T}{\partial r}\right) + \frac{\partial}{\partial z}\left(k\frac{\partial T}{\partial z}\right) + Q_{\mathrm{m}} \quad (8.1d)
$$

Q_{m} (W/cm^3) is the volumetric metabolic rate of heat generation of the unfrozen tissue. Equation (8.1d) has a variable coefficient that forms a singularity ($1/r$ for $r = 0$) and nonlinear coefficients resulting from temperature-dependent physical properties ($C(T), k(T)$).

The probe tip is placed so that

$$T(r = 0, z = z_{\mathrm{p}}, t) = T_{\mathrm{p}}(t) \tag{8.1e}$$

where T_{p} is the probe tip temperature. At all other points (other than $r = 0, z = z_{\mathrm{p}}$), the temperature is calculated by the solution of eq. (8.1d).

As discussed by Deng et al. [1], the physical properties of eq. (8.1d) are programmed as a function of T, that is, $C = C(T), k = k(T)$ to account for the differences of these properties for frozen and unfrozen tissues.

$$C(T) = \begin{cases} C_{\mathrm{f}}, & T < T_{\mathrm{ml}} \\ \dfrac{Q_{\mathrm{l}}}{T_{\mathrm{mu}} - T_{\mathrm{ml}}} + \dfrac{C_{\mathrm{f}} + C_{\mathrm{u}}}{2}, & T_{\mathrm{ml}} \leq T \leq T_{\mathrm{mu}} \\ C_{\mathrm{u}}, & T > T_{\mathrm{mu}} \end{cases} \tag{8.1f}$$

$$k(T) = \begin{cases} k_{\mathrm{f}}, & T < T_{\mathrm{ml}} \\ \dfrac{k_{\mathrm{f}} + k_{\mathrm{u}}}{2}, & T_{\mathrm{ml}} \leq T \leq T_{\mathrm{mu}} \\ k_{\mathrm{u}}, & T > T_{\mathrm{mu}} \end{cases} \tag{8.1g}$$

In eqs. (8.1f) and (8.1g), $T_{\mathrm{ml}}, T_{\mathrm{mu}}$ are the temperatures at which a phase transition between frozen and unfrozen tissues takes place; the subscripts l, u in these temperatures refer to lower and upper, respectively, whereas f in $C_{\mathrm{f}}, k_{\mathrm{f}}$ refers to frozen and u in $C_{\mathrm{u}}, k_{\mathrm{u}}$ refers to unfrozen.

Additionally, the volumetric metabolic rate of heat generation of the unfrozen tissue, Q_{m}, is given by

$$Q_{\mathrm{m}}(T) = \begin{cases} 0, & T < T_{\mathrm{mu}} \\ Q_{\mathrm{mu}}, & T > T_{\mathrm{mu}} \end{cases} \tag{8.1h}$$

where Q_{mu} is a constant (for the unfrozen tissue).

Eq. (8.1d) is first order in t and second order in r and z. It, therefore, requires one IC in t and two BCs in r and z. We take these auxiliary conditions to be

$$T(r, z, t = 0) = T_0 \tag{8.2}$$

$$\frac{\partial T(r = r_p, z, t)}{\partial r} = \frac{\partial T(r = r_c, z, t)}{\partial r} = 0, \quad 0 \le z \le z_p \tag{8.3a,b}$$

$$\frac{\partial T(r = 0, z, t)}{\partial r} = \frac{\partial T(r = r_c, z, t)}{\partial r} = 0, \quad z_p < z \le z_c \tag{8.3c,d}$$

$$T(r, z = 0, t) = T_s; \quad \frac{\partial T(r, z = z_c, t)}{\partial z} = 0 \tag{8.3e,f}$$

where

Parameter	Interpretation
T_0	tissue initial temperature (°C)
T_s	tissue surface temperature (°C)
r_p	radius of the probe (cm)
r_c	radius of the cryosurgery domain (cm)
z_p	length of the probe (cm)
z_c	length of the cryosurgery domain (cm)

The BCs in r, eqs. (8.3a)–(8.3d) are stated in two parts (refer to Fig. 8.1). But because the probe radius is small compared to the grid spacing in r, we will take $r_p \approx 0$, so that BCs (8.3a) and (8.3c) are used at $r = 0$. In other words, BCs (8.3a), (8.3b), (8.3c) and (8.3d) constitute two BCs at $r = 0$ reflecting symmetry around $r = 0$, and two BCs at $r = r_c$ reflecting no variation with r at the outer boundary.

Eqs. (8.3b), (8.3d), and (8.3f) are insulated (zero heat flux, zero conduction) BCs. Eq. (8.2e) specifies a constant surface temperature T_s at $z = 0$.

To repeat, at the probe tip ($r = 0, z = z_p$), $T(r, z, t)$ is taken as $T(r = 0, z = z_p, t) = T_p(t)$ where $T_p(t)$ is the probe temperature, typically a constant. This is programmed as $\partial T(r = 0, z = z_p, t)/\partial t = 0$ for a constant probe tip temperature with an IC of T_p (note this is a derivative in t, not r).

The MOL programming of the model consisting of eqs. (8.1d)–(8.1h), (8.2), and (8.3) is considered in the following section.

8.3 Method of Lines Analysis

To start with the simplest case for the MOL analysis, we consider $r_p \approx 0$ as mentioned previously, that is, the probe has a diameter that is small enough so that the probe is essentially located entirely at $r = 0$. The case of a larger probe diameter will be discussed subsequently. The principal complications in analyzing the PDE, eqs. (8.1d)–(8.1h) are as follows:

1. The $1/r$ singularity in eq. (8.1d).
2. The single point probe temperature of eq. (8.1e).
3. The variable properties of eqs. (8.1f)–(8.1h).

The following routines provide an explanation of how these three requirements are programmed.

8.3.1 ODE Routine

The MOL ODE routine, `cryo_1`, is in Listing 8.1.

```
  cryo_1=function(t,u,parms){
#
# Function cryo_1 computes the t derivative vector of
#    T(r,z,t)
#
# 1D vector to 2D matrix
   T=matrix(0,nrow=nr,ncol=nz);
  Tt=matrix(0,nrow=nr,ncol=nz);
  for(i in 1:nr){
  for(j in 1:nz){
    T[i,j]=u[(i-1)*nz+j];
  }
  }
#
# ODEs at grid points in r and z
  for(i in 1:nr){
  for(j in 1:nz){
#
#    r=0
    if(i==1){
```

```
#
#     z=0
      if(j==1){
        T[1,1]=Ts;
        Tt[1,1]=0;
#
#     z=zp
      }else if(j==np){
        T[1,np]=Tp;
        Tt[1,np]=0;
#
#     z=zc
      }else if(j==nz){
        term1=4*kc(T[1,nz])*(T[2,nz]-T[1,nz])/drs;
        term2=2*kc(T[1,nz])*(T[1,nz-1]-T[1,nz])/dzs;
        Tt[1,nz]=1/Cp(T[1,nz])*(term1+term2
           +Qm(T[1,nz]));
#
#     z ne 0, zp, zc
      }else{
        term1=4*kc(T[1,j])*(T[2,j]-T[1,j])/drs;
        term2=  kc(T[1,j])*(T[1,j+1]-2*T[1,j]+T[1,j-1])
           /dzs;
        term3= dkc(T[1,j])*((T[1,j+1]-T[1,j-1])/(2*dz))^2;
        Tt[1,j]=1/Cp(T[1,j])*(term1+term2+term3
           +Qm(T[1,j]));
      }
#
#   r=rc
    }else if(i==nr){
#
#     z=0
      if(j==1){
        T[nr,1]=Ts;
        Tt[nr,1]=0;
#
#     z=zc
      }else if(j==nz){
        Tnrp1=T[nr-1,nz];
        term1=  kc(T[nr,nz])*(Tnrp1-2*T[nr,nz]+T[nr-1,nz])
           /drs;
```

```
          term2=2*kc(T[nr,nz])*(T[nr,nz]-T[nr,nz-1])/dzs;
          Tt[nr,nz]=1/Cp(T[nr,nz])*(term1+term2
             +Qm(T[nr,nz]));
#
#       z ne 0, zc
        }else{
          Tnrp1=T[nr-1,j];
          term1= kc(T[nr,j])*(Tnrp1-2*T[nr,j]+T[nr-1,j])
             /drs;
          term2= kc(T[nr,j])*(T[nr,j+1]-2*T[nr,j]+T[nr,j-1])
             /dzs;
          term3=dkc(T[nr,j])*(T[nr,j+1]-T[nr,j-1])/(2*dz);
          Tt[nr,j]=1/Cp(T[nr,j])*(term1+term2+term3
             +Qm(T[nr,j]));
        }
#
#     r ne 0, rc
      }else{
#
#       z=0
        if(j==1){
          T[i,1]=Ts;
          Tt[i,1]=0;
#
#       z=zc
        }else if(j==nz){
          term1= kc(T[i,nz])*(T[i+1,nz]-2*T[i,nz]+T[i-1,nz])
             /drs;
          term2=dkc(T[i,nz])*((T[i+1,nz]-T[i-1,nz])
             /(2*dr))^2;
          term3=(1/r[i])*kc(T[i,nz])*(T[i+1,nz]-T[i-1,nz])
             /(2*dr);
          term4=2*kc(T[i,nz])*(T[i,nz-1]-T[i,nz])/dzs;
          Tt[i,nz]=1/Cp(T[i,nz])*(term1+term2+term3+term4
             +Qm(T[i,nz]));
#
#       z ne 0, zc
        }else{
          term1= kc(T[i,j])*(T[i+1,j]-2*T[i,j]+T[i-1,j])
             /drs;
          term2=dkc(T[i,j])*((T[i+1,j]-T[i-1,j])/(2*dr))^2;
```

```
        term3=(1/r[i])*kc(T[i,j])*(T[i+1,j]-T[i-1,j])
           /(2*dr);
        term4= kc(T[i,j])*(T[i,j+1]-2*T[i,j]+T[i,j-1])
           /dzs;
        term5=dkc(T[i,j])*((T[i,j+1]-T[i,j-1])/(2*dz))^2;
        Tt[i,j]=1/Cp(T[i,j])*(term1+term2+term3+term4
           +term5+Qm(T[i,j]));
      }
    }
#
# Next i
  }
#
# Next j
  }
#
# 2D matrix to 1D vector
  ut=rep(0,nr*nz);
  for(i in 1:nr){
  for(j in 1:nz){
    ut[(i-1)*nz+j]=Tt[i,j];
  }
  }
#
# Increment calls to cryo_1
  ncall <<- ncall+1;
#
# Return derivative vector
  return(list(c(ut)));
}
```

Listing 8.1 ODE routine pde_1 for eqs. (8.1d)–(8.1h).

We can note the following details about Listing 8.1.

- The function is defined.

```
  cryo_1=function(t,u,parms){
#
# Function cryo_1 computes the t derivative vector of
#    T(r,z,t)
```

u is the vector of length nr*nz where nr and nz, the number of points in r and z, respectively, are defined in the main program to be discussed subsequently. Here, we are making use of an R feature in which variables defined numerically in a superior routine, in this case the main program, are available in a subordinate routine, in this case cryo_1, without any special designation (e.g., they do not have to be declared global or common).

- The input vector u is placed in a 2D matrix, T.

```
#
# 1D vector to 2D matrix
   T=matrix(0,nrow=nr,ncol=nz);
  Tt=matrix(0,nrow=nr,ncol=nz);
  for(i in 1:nr){
  for(j in 1:nz){
    T[i,j]=u[(i-1)*nz+j];
  }
  }
```

T and Tt are first declared (preallocated) with the matrix utility. Tt is a nr $\times$ nz matrix that will contain the computed derivative in t from eq. (8.1d), that is, $\partial T(r,z,t)/\partial t$ at a particular value of t.

T[i,j] is defined numerically by two for's with indices i and j that refer to a particular r and z, respectively. The range of the indices is $1 \le$ i $\le$ nr, $1 \le$ j $\le$ nz, $1 \le$ (i-1)*nz+j $\le$ nr*nz (the reader should verify the last range as the for's are executed corresponding to i=1,j=1 to i=nr,j=nz).

The nr*nz ODEs are programmed within two for's.

```
#
# ODEs at grid points in r and z
  for(i in 1:nr){
  for(j in 1:nz){
#
#   r=0
    if(i==1){
```

corresponding to the (r,z) domain $0 \le r \le r_c$, $0 \le z \le z_c$ where r_c and z_c are the lengths of the domain in r and z, respectively.

Initially, the ODEs along the radial centerline $r = 0$ (with `i=1`) are programmed, that is, for $r = 0$, $0 \le z \le z_c$.

- BC (8.3e) is programmed corresponding to $r = 0, z = 0$ (`i=1,j=1`).

```
#
#       z=0
        if(j==1){
          T[1,1]=Ts;
          Tt[1,1]=0;
```

As $T(r = 0, z = 0, t)$ is a constant, T_s, its derivative in t, `Tt`, is zero (this is the first of the `nr*nz=6*11=66` ODEs).

- $T(r = 0, z = z_p, t) = T_p$ is programmed according to eq. (8.1e) where z_p is the length of the cryoprobe and T_p is the temperature of the probe tip.

```
#
#       z=zp
        }else if(j==np){
          T[1,np]=Tp;
          Tt[1,np]=0;
```

In other words, this is how the low temperature in the cryosurgery is applied. This implies that the region (e.g., tumor) to be treated is located near $r = 0, z = z_p$. In this case, the index in z is defined numerically in the main program as `j=np` (corresponding to $z = z_c/2$ but any other value of the index `j` could be used to locate the probe tip). Also, because T_p is constant, the derivative in t, `Tt`, is zero.

- The ODE at $r = 0, z = z_c$ is programmed corresponding to the indices (`i=1,j=nz`).

```
#
#       z=zc
        }else if(j==nz){
          term1=4*kc(T[1,nz])*(T[2,nz]-T[1,nz])/drs;
          term2=2*kc(T[1,nz])*(T[1,nz-1]-T[1,nz])/dzs;
          Tt[1,nz]=1/Cp(T[1,nz])*(term1+term2
             +Qm(T[1,nz]));
```

Note the use of the subscripts (`1,nz`) corresponding to $r = 0, z_c$ and the use of the function `kc` for $k(T)$ and `Cp` for $C_p(T)$. These functions are discussed subsequently.

Some additional explanation for the preceding coding is required.

— The derivative in r of eq. (8.1d)

$$\frac{1}{r}\frac{\partial}{\partial r}\left(rk\frac{\partial T}{\partial r}\right)$$

is programmed as `term1`. From differentiation of a product of three functions (considering $k = k(T)$),

$$\frac{1}{r}\frac{\partial}{\partial r}\left(rk\frac{\partial T}{\partial r}\right) = k\frac{\partial^2 T}{\partial r^2} + \frac{dk}{dT}\left(\frac{\partial T}{\partial r}\right)^2 + \frac{1}{r}k\frac{\partial T}{\partial r} \tag{8.4a}$$

The third term of eq. (8.4a) is indeterminate at $r = 0$ because from BC (8.3c) with $z = z_c$, $\dfrac{\partial T(r = 0,\ z = z_c, t)}{\partial r} = 0$. This indeterminate form can be resolved with l'Hospital's rule (differentiating numerator and denominator with respect to r).

$$\lim_{r \to 0} \frac{1}{r}k\frac{\partial T}{\partial r} = k\frac{\partial^2 T}{\partial r^2} \tag{8.4b}$$

Thus, from eq. (8.4b), eq. (8.4a) becomes

$$\frac{1}{r}\frac{\partial}{\partial r}\left(rk\frac{\partial T}{\partial r}\right) = 2k\frac{\partial^2 T}{\partial r^2} + \frac{dk}{dT}\left(\frac{\partial T}{\partial r}\right)^2$$

or with BC (8.3c)

$$\frac{1}{r}\frac{\partial}{\partial r}\left(rk\frac{\partial T}{\partial r}\right) = 2k\frac{\partial^2 T}{\partial r^2} \tag{8.4c}$$

The three-point centered FD approximation of the second derivative term in eq. (8.4c) is

$$2k\frac{\partial^2 T}{\partial r^2} \approx 2k\frac{T(r = dr, z = z_c, t) - 2T(r = 0, z = z_c, t) + T(r = -dr, z = z_c, t)}{dr^2} \tag{8.4d}$$

where dr is the MOL grid spacing in r. $T(r=-dr, z=z_c, t)$ is a fictitious value (outside $0 \le r \le r_c$) that can be evaluated from BC (8.3c) with $z=z_c$, that is,

$$\frac{\partial T(r=0, z=z_c, t)}{\partial r}=0$$

which can be approximated with a two-point centered FD as

$$\frac{\partial T(r=0, z=z_c, t)}{\partial r} \approx \frac{T(r=dr, z=z_c, t) - T(r=-dr, z=z_c, t)}{2dr}=0$$

The fictitious value is, therefore, $T(r=-dr, z=z_c, t)= T(r=dr, z=z_c, t)$ and eq. (8.4d) is

$$2k\frac{\partial^2 T}{\partial r^2} \approx 4k\frac{T(r=dr, z=z_c, t)-T(r=0, z=z_c, t)}{dr^2} \tag{8.4e}$$

which is programmed as

```
term1=4*kc(T[1,nz])*(T[2,nz]-T[1,nz])/drs;
```

Note the dk/dT term in eq. (8.4a) is not used because $\partial T(r= 0, z, t)/\partial r = 0$ (from BC (8.3c)).

— The derivative in z of eq. (8.1d)

$$\frac{\partial}{\partial z}\left(k\frac{\partial T}{\partial z}\right)$$

is programmed in a similar manner. From differentiation of a product of two functions (considering $k=k(T)$),

$$\frac{\partial}{\partial z}\left(k\frac{\partial T}{\partial z}\right)=k\frac{\partial^2 T}{\partial z^2}+\frac{dk}{dT}\left(\frac{\partial T}{\partial z}\right)^2 \tag{8.5a}$$

or with BC (8.3f)

$$\frac{\partial}{\partial z}\left(k\frac{\partial T}{\partial z}\right)=k\frac{\partial^2 T}{\partial z^2} \tag{8.5b}$$

The three-point centered FD approximation of this result is

$$k\frac{\partial^2 T}{\partial z^2} \approx k\frac{T(r=0,z=z_c+dz,t)-2T(r=0,z=z_c,t) + T(r=0,z=z_c-dz,t)}{dz^2} \tag{8.5c}$$

where dz is the MOL grid spacing in z. $T(r=0,z=z_c+dz,t)$ is a fictitious value (outside $0 \le z \le z_c$) which can be evaluated from BC (8.3f) (with $r=0$), that is,

$$\frac{\partial T(r=0,z=z_c,t)}{\partial z} = 0$$

can be approximated with a two-point centered FD as

$$\frac{\partial T(r=0,z=z_c,t)}{\partial z} \approx \frac{T(r=0,z=z_c+dz,t) - T(r=0,z=z_c-dz,t)}{2dz} = 0$$

The fictitious value is therefore $T(r=0,z=z_c+dz,t) = T(r=0,z=z_c-dz,t)$ and eq. (8.5c) is

$$2k\frac{\partial^2 T}{\partial z^2} \approx 2k\frac{T(r=0,z=z_c-dz,t)-T(r=0,z=z_c,t)}{dz^2} \tag{8.5d}$$

which is programmed as

```
term2=2*kc(T[1,nz])*(T[1,nz-1]-T[1,nz])/dzs;
```

Note the dk/dT term in eq. (8.5a) is not used because $\partial T(r,z=z_c,t)/\partial z = 0$ (from BC (8.3f)).

Eq. (8.1d) at $r=0, z=z_c$ is then programmed as

```
Tt[1,nz]=1/Cp(T[1,nz])*(term1+term2+Qm(T[1,nz]));
```

- The ODEs at $r=0, z \neq 0, z_c, z_p$ are programmed as

```
#
#     z ne 0, zp, zc
      }else{
        term1=4*kc(T[1,j])*(T[2,j]-T[1,j])/drs;
```

```
    term2=  kc(T[1,j])*(T[1,j+1]-2*T[1,j]+T
       [1,j-1])/dzs;
    term3= dkc(T[1,j])*((T[1,j+1]-T[1,j-1])
       /(2*dz))^2;
    Tt[1,j]=1/Cp(T[1,j])*(term1+term2+term3
       +Qm(T[1,j]));
}
```

Note the use of the subscripts `1,j` corresponding to $r = 0, z$, and the use of the function `dkc` for dk/dT in eq. (8.5a) (this function is discussed subsequently). Some additional explanation is required.

— The radial derivative in eq. (8.1d) is similar to eq. (8.4e) but with z in place of $z = z_c$ (or `j` in place of `nz`)

$$2k\frac{\partial^2 T}{\partial r^2} \approx 4k\frac{T(r = dr, z, t) - T(r = 0, z, t)}{dr^2} \tag{8.6a}$$

and is programmed as

```
term1=4*kc(T[1,j])*(T[2,j]-T[1,j])/drs;
```

— The programming of the derivative in z in eq. (8.1d) is based on the following FD approximations. For

$$k\frac{\partial^2 T}{\partial z^2}$$

in eq. (8.5a), the FD approximation is

$$k\frac{\begin{array}{c}T(r = 0, z = z + dz, t) - 2T(r = 0, z, t)\\ + T(r = 0, z = z - dz, t)\end{array}}{dz^2} \tag{8.6b}$$

and is programmed as

```
term2=kc(T[1,j])*(T[1,j+1]-2*T[1,j]+T[1,j-1])
   /dzs;
```

For

$$\frac{dk}{dT}\left(\frac{\partial T}{\partial z}\right)^2$$

in eq. (8.5a), the FD approximation is

$$\frac{dk}{dT}\left(\frac{T(r=0,z=z+dz,t)-T(r=0,z=z-dz,t)}{2dz}\right)^2 \tag{8.6c}$$

and is programmed as

```
term3= dkc(T[1,j])*((T[1,j+1]-T[1,j-1])
   /(2*dz))^2;
```

The programming of eq. (8.1d) (for $r = 0$) is then

```
Tt[1,j]=1/Cp(T[1,j])*(term1+term2+term3
   +Qm(T[1,j]));
```

This completes the programming of the nz ODEs at $r = 0$.

To continue the discussion of cryo_1 of Listing 8.1,

- The programming of the nz ODEs at $r = dr, 2dr, \ldots$ or i=2,3,... is as follows:

```
#
#    r ne 0, rc
     }else{
#
#      z=0
       if(j==1){
         T[i,1]=Ts;
         Tt[i,1]=0;
```

BC (8.3e) is programmed as before corresponding to $r, z = 0$ (i,j=1).

- The programming at $r, z = z_c$ is

```
#
#      z=zc
       }else if(j==nz){
         term1= kc(T[i,nz])*(T[i+1,nz]-2*T[i,nz]+T
            [i-1,nz])/drs;
         term2=dkc(T[i,nz])*((T[i+1,nz]-T[i-1,nz])
```

```
        /(2*dr))^2;
    term3=(1/r[i])*kc(T[i,nz])*(T[i+1,nz]-T
        [i-1,nz])/(2*dr);
    term4=2*kc(T[i,nz])*(T[i,nz-1]-T[i,nz])/dzs;
    Tt[i,nz]=1/Cp(T[i,nz])*(term1+term2+term3
        +term4+Qm(T[i,nz]));
```

Some additional explanation is required.

— The second derivative $\partial^2 T(r, z = z_c, t)/\partial r^2$ in eq. (8.4a) is approximated as

$$\frac{T(r = r + dr, z = z_c, t) - 2T(r = r, z = z_c, t) + T(r = r - dr, z = z_c, t)}{dr^2}$$

and is programmed as

```
term1= kc(T[i,nz])*(T[i+1,nz]-2*T[i,nz]+
    T[i-1,nz])/drs;
```

— The dk/dT term in eq. (8.4a), $dk/dT[\partial T(r, z = z_c, t)/\partial r)]^2$, is programmed as

```
term2=dkc(T[i,nz])*((T[i+1,nz]-T[i-1,nz])
    /(2*dr))^2;
```

— The variable coefficient term in eq. (8.4a), $(1/r)k\partial T(r, z = z_c, t)/\partial r$, is programmed as

```
term3=(1/r[i])*kc(T[i,nz])*(T[i+1,nz]-T[i-1,nz])
    /(2*dr);
```

— The second derivative $\partial^2 T(r, z = z_c, t)/\partial z^2$ with BC (8.3f) in eq. (8.5a) is programmed as

```
term4=2*kc(T[i,nz])*(T[i,nz-1]-T[i,nz])/dzs;
```

— Equation (8.1d) at $(r, z = z_c)$ or `i,j=nz` is programmed as

```
Tt[i,nz]=1/Cp(T[i,nz])*(term1+term2+term3+term4
    +Qm(T[i,nz]));
```

Finally, the programming of eq. (8.1d) at the interior points, that is, $r \neq 0, r_c, z \neq 0, z_c$ or `i,j` is

```
#
#      z ne 0, zc
       }else{
         term1= kc(T[i,j])*(T[i+1,j]-2*T[i,j]+T[i-1,j])
            /drs;
         term2=dkc(T[i,j])*((T[i+1,j]-T[i-1,j])
            /(2*dr))^2;
         term3=(1/r[i])*kc(T[i,j])*(T[i+1,j]-T[i-1,j])
            /(2*dr);
         term4= kc(T[i,j])*(T[i,j+1]-2*T[i,j]+T[i,j-1])
            /dzs;
         term5=dkc(T[i,j])*((T[i,j+1]-T[i,j-1])
            /(2*dz))^2;
         Tt[i,j]=1/Cp(T[i,j])*(term1+term2+term3+term4
            +term5+Qm(T[i,j]));
       }
     }
```

Some additional explanation is required.

— The second derivative $\partial^2 T(r,z,t)/\partial^2 r$ in eq. (8.4a) is programmed as

```
term1= kc(T[i,j])*(T[i+1,j]-2*T[i,j]+T[i-1,j])
   /drs;
```

— The dk/dT term in eq. (8.4a) is programmed as

```
term2=dkc(T[i,j])*((T[i+1,j]-T[i-1,j])
   /(2*dr))^2;
```

— The $1/r$ term in eq. (8.4a) is programmed as

```
term3=(1/r[i])*kc(T[i,j])*(T[i+1,j]-T[i-1,j])
   /(2*dr);
```

— The second derivative $\partial^2 T(r,z,t)/\partial^2 z$ in eq. (8.5a) is programmed as

```
term4= kc(T[i,j])*(T[i,j+1]-2*T[i,j]+T[i,j-1])
   /dzs;
```

— The dk/dT term in eq. (8.5a) is programmed as

```
term5=dkc(T[i,j])*((T[i,j+1]-T[i,j-1])
   /(2*dz))^2;
```

— Then, eq. (8.1d) is programmed as

```
Tt[i,j]=1/Cp(T[i,j])*(term1+term2+term3
   +term4+term5+Qm(T[i,j]));
```

- This completes the programming of all of the $(nr)(nz) = (6)(11) = 66$ derivatives in t (in array `Tt`), so the two `for`'s in r and z can be concluded.

```
#
# Next i
  }
#
# Next j
  }
```

- The 2D matrix `Tt` is placed in the 1D vector `ut` for use by the ODE integrator `lsodes` called by the main program considered subsequently.

```
#
# 2D matrix to 1D vector
  ut=rep(0,nr*nz);
  for(i in 1:nr){
  for(j in 1:nz){
    ut[(i-1)*nz+j]=Tt[i,j];
  }
  }
```

Note that this coding is essentially the reverse of the `u` to `T` coding at the beginning of `cryo_1` which ensures that each dependent variable in `u` has a derivative placed in the corresponding position in `ut`. This one-to-one correspondence is essential for the correct integration of the `66` ODEs.

- The counter for the calls to `cryo_1` is incremented and returned to the main program with `<<-`.

```
#
# Increment calls to cryo_1
  ncall <<- ncall+1;
```

- The derivative vector `ut` is returned from `cryo_1` as a list, which is required by the R ODE integrators such as `lsodes`.

```
#
# Return derivative vector
  return(list(c(ut)));
}
```

  `c` is the R vector operator. The final `}` concludes `cryo_1`.

This completes the programming of `cryo_1`. As the functions `Cp, kc, dkc, Qm` are called from `cryo_1`, they are considered next.

8.3.2 Physical Property Routines

The programming of eq. (8.1f) is in function `Cp`.

```
  Cp=function(T){
#
# Parameters
  Tml=-8;Tmu=-1;Cf=1.8;Cu=3.6;Ql=250;
#
# Variable heat capacity
  if(T<Tml){
    Cp=Cf;
  }else if((Tml<=T)&(T<=Tmu)){
    Cp=Ql/(Tmu-Tml)+(Cf+Cu)/2;
  }else if(T>Tmu){
    Cp=Cu;
  }
  return(c(Cp));
  }
```

Listing 8.2 Function `Cp` for the specific heat in eq. (8.1d).

This coding is essentially self-explanatory by comparison with eq. (8.1f). The parameters for the calculation of the specific heat are defined numerically at the beginning of the routine. The temperature interval for the phase transition from frozen to unfrozen is `Tml-Tmu` (these temperatures are slightly lower than the freezing point of water, $0^\circ C$). Note that `Cp` is returned as a 1-vector (scalar) with the R `c` vector utility.

The programming of eq. (8.1g), with a modification, is in function `kc` (Listing 8.3).

```
  kc=function(T){
#
# Parameters
  Tml=-8;Tmu=-1;kf=0.02;ku=0.005;
#
# Variable conductivity
  if(T<Tml){
    kc=kf;
  }else if((Tml<=T)&(T<=Tmu)){
    kc=kf+(T-Tml)/(Tmu-Tml)*(ku-kf);
  }else if(T>Tmu){
    kc=ku;
  }
  return(c(kc));
  }
```

Listing 8.3 Function `kc` for the thermal conductivity in eq. (8.1d).

Again, the parameters for the calculation of the thermal conductivity are defined numerically at the beginning of the routine. The temperature interval for the phase transition from frozen to unfrozen is `Tml-Tmu`. Within this interval, `kc` varies linearly with temperature

```
    kc=kf+(T-Tml)/(Tmu-Tml)*(ku-kf);
```

rather than as an average value as in eq. (8.1g). This linear function with slope `(ku-kf)/(Tmu-Tml)` provides the derivative dk/dT required in eqs. (8.4a) and (8.5a). Note that the linear function has the end points

```
(T=Tml=-8,kc=kf=0.02), (T=Tmu=-1,kc=ku=0.005),
```

corresponding to the frozen and unfrozen states, respectively.

The programming of the derivative dk/dT is in function dkc (listing 8.4).

```
  dkc=function(T){
#
# Parameters
  Tml=-8;Tmu=-1;kf=0.02;ku=0.005;
#
# Variable conductivity
  if(T<Tml){
    dkc=0;
  }else if((Tml<=T)&(T<=Tmu)){
    dkc=(ku-kf)/(Tmu-Tml);
  }else if(T>Tmu){
    dkc=0;
  }
  return(c(dkc));
  }
```

Listing 8.4 Function dkc for the derivative of the thermal conductivity, dk/dT, in eqs. (8.4a) and (8.5a).

The coding in dkc follows immediately from kc in Listing 8.3. Note the slope of the linear function, dkc=(ku-kf)/(Tmu-Tml).

The programming of eq. (8.1h) is in function Qm (Listing 8.5).

```
  Qm=function(T){
#
# Parameters
  Tmu=-1;Qmu=0.0042;
#
# Variable source
  if(T<=Tmu){
    Qm=0;
  }else if(T>Tmu){
    Qm=Qmu;
  }
```

```
return(c(Qm));
}
```

Listing 8.5 Function Qm for the source term in eq. (8.1d).

This coding follows immediately from eq. (8.1h). Qm=0 in the frozen state reflects no heat generation from metabolism. Qm=Qmu in the unfrozen state reflects positive volumetric heat generation from metabolism.

This completes the programming of the temperature-dependent physical properties in eq. (8.1d). We now consider the main program that calls cryo_1 and, in turn, Cp, kc, dkc, Qm.

8.3.3 Main Program

```
#
# Access ODE integrator
  library("deSolve");
#
# Access functions for numerical solutions
  setwd("c:/R/bme_pde/chap8");
  source("cryo_1.R");
  source("kc.R");
  source("Cp.R");
  source("Qm.R");
  source("dkc.R");
#
# Model parameters
    rc=5;  zc=10;  Ts=37; Tp=-196; Qmt=0.0042;
  Cb=3.6; Cu=3.6; Cf=1.8; kf=0.02; ku=0.005; Ql=250;
  Tml=-8; Tmu=-1;
#
# Radial grid
  nr=6;dr=rc/(nr-1);drs=dr^2;
  r=seq(from=0,to=rc,by=dr);
#
# Axial grid
  nz=11;np=6;
  dz=zc/(nz-1);dzs=dz^2;
  z=seq(from=0,to=zc,by=dz);
```

```
#
# Grid in t
  nout=5;tf=120;
  tout=seq(from=0,to=tf,by=tf/(nout-1));
#
# Display selected parameters
  cat(sprintf(
    "\n\n   nr = %2d   np = %2d   nz = %2d\n",nr,np,nz));
#
# Initial condition
  u0=rep(0,nr*nz);T0=Ts;
  for(i in 1:nr){
  for(j in 1:nz){
    u0[(i-1)*nz+j]=T0;
  }
  }
  ncall=0;
#
# ODE integration
  out=lsodes(y=u0,times=tout,func=cryo_1,parms=NULL);
  nrow(out)
  ncol(out)
#
# Calls to ODE routine
  cat(sprintf("\n\n   ncall = %5d\n\n",ncall));
#
# Plot z profiles
  T_zplot1=matrix(0,nrow=nz,ncol=nout);
  T_zplot2=matrix(0,nrow=nz,ncol=nout);
  T_zplot3=matrix(0,nrow=nz,ncol=nout);
  T_zplot4=matrix(0,nrow=nz,ncol=nout);
  T_zplot5=matrix(0,nrow=nz,ncol=nout);
  T_zplot6=matrix(0,nrow=nz,ncol=nout);
  for(it in 1:nout){
    for(j in 1:nz){
      T_zplot1[j,it]=out[it,     j+1];
      T_zplot2[j,it]=out[it,  nz+j+1];
      T_zplot3[j,it]=out[it,2*nz+j+1];
      T_zplot4[j,it]=out[it,3*nz+j+1];
      T_zplot5[j,it]=out[it,4*nz+j+1];
      T_zplot6[j,it]=out[it,5*nz+j+1];
```

```
    }
      T_zplot1[np,it]=Tp;
      T_zplot1[1,it] =Ts;
      T_zplot2[1,it] =Ts;
      T_zplot3[1,it] =Ts;
      T_zplot4[1,it] =Ts;
      T_zplot5[1,it] =Ts;
      T_zplot6[1,it] =Ts;
  }
#
# Automatic vertical scaling for each plot
  par(mfrow=c(3,2));
  matplot(x=z,y=T_zplot1,type="l",xlab="z",
          ylab="T(r=0,z,t)",xlim=c(0,z[nz]),lty=1,
          main="T(r=0,z,t),t=0,30,...,120",lwd=2);
  matplot(x=z,y=T_zplot2,type="l",xlab="z",
          ylab="T(r=1,z,t)",xlim=c(0,z[nz]),lty=1,
          main="T(r=1,z,t),t=0,30,...,120",lwd=2);
  matplot(x=z,y=T_zplot3,type="l",xlab="z",
          ylab="T(r=2,z,t)",xlim=c(0,z[nz]),lty=1,
          main="T(r=2,z,t),t=0,30,...,120",lwd=2);
  matplot(x=z,y=T_zplot4,type="l",xlab="z",
          ylab="T(r=3,z,t)",xlim=c(0,z[nz]),lty=1,
          main="T(r=3,z,t),t=0,30,...,120",lwd=2);
  matplot(x=z,y=T_zplot5,type="l",xlab="z",
          ylab="T(r=4,z,t)",xlim=c(0,z[nz]),lty=1,
          main="T(r=4,z,t),t=0,30,...,120",lwd=2);
  matplot(x=z,y=T_zplot6,type="l",xlab="z",
          ylab="T(r=5,z,t)",xlim=c(0,z[nz]),lty=1,
          main="T(r=5,z,t),t=0,30,...,120",lwd=2);
#
# Vertical scale set as -200 <= T <= 40
  par(mfrow=c(3,2));
  matplot(x=z,y=T_zplot1,type="l",xlab="z",
          ylab="T(r=0,z,t)",xlim=c(0,z[nz]),lty=1,
          main="T(r=0,z,t),t=0,30,...,120",lwd=2,
          ylim=c(-200,40));
  matplot(x=z,y=T_zplot2,type="l",xlab="z",
          ylab="T(r=1,z,t)",xlim=c(0,z[nz]),lty=1,
          main="T(r=1,z,t),t=0,30,...,120",lwd=2,
          ylim=c(-200,40));
```

```
matplot(x=z,y=T_zplot3,type="l",xlab="z",
        ylab="T(r=2,z,t)",xlim=c(0,z[nz]),lty=1,
        main="T(r=2,z,t),t=0,30,...,120",lwd=2,
        ylim=c(-200,40));
matplot(x=z,y=T_zplot4,type="l",xlab="z",
        ylab="T(r=3,z,t)",xlim=c(0,z[nz]),lty=1,
        main="T(r=3,z,t),t=0,30,...,120",lwd=2,
        ylim=c(-200,40));
matplot(x=z,y=T_zplot5,type="l",xlab="z",
        ylab="T(r=4,z,t)",xlim=c(0,z[nz]),lty=1,
        main="T(r=4,z,t),t=0,30,...,120",lwd=2,
        ylim=c(-200,40));
matplot(x=z,y=T_zplot6,type="l",xlab="z",
        ylab="T(r=5,z,t)",xlim=c(0,z[nz]),lty=1,
        main="T(r=5,z,t),t=0,30,...,120",lwd=2,
        ylim=c(-200,40));
```

Listing 8.6 Main program for eqs. (8.1d)–(8.1h).

We can note the following details about Listing 8.6.

- The R ODE integrators in `deSolve` and the various routines discussed previously are accessed.

```
#
# Access ODE integrator
  library("deSolve");
#
# Access functions for numerical solutions
  setwd("c:/R/bme_pde/chap8");
  source("cryo_1.R");
  source("kc.R");
  source("Cp.R");
  source("Qm.R");
  source("dkc.R");
```

  Note the forward slash / rather than the usual backslash \ in the `setwd` (set working directory).
- The model parameters are defined numerically [1].

```
#
# Model parameters
```

```
    rc=5;  zc=10;  Ts=37; Tp=-196; Qmt=0.0042;
  Cb=3.6; Cu=3.6; Cf=1.8; kf=0.02; ku=0.005; Ql=250;
  Tml=-8; Tmu=-1;
```

- A grid in r with spacing `dr=1` is defined for the six points $r = 0, 1, \ldots, 5$.

```
#
# Radial grid
  nr=6;dr=rc/(nr-1);drs=dr^2;
  r=seq(from=0,to=rc,by=dr);
```

- A grid in z with spacing `dz=1` is defined for the 11 points $z = 0, 1, \ldots, 10$.

```
#
# Axial grid
  nz=11;np=6;
  dz=zc/(nz-1);dzs=dz^2;
  z=seq(from=0,to=zc,by=dz);
```

- A grid in t with spacing `30` is defined for the output five points $t = 0, 30, \ldots, 120$.

```
#
# Grid in t
  nout=5;tf=120;
  tout=seq(from=0,to=tf,by=tf/(nout-1));
```

- Selected parameters are displayed.

```
#
# Display selected parameters
  cat(sprintf(
    "\n\n    nr = %2d    np = %2d    nz = %2d\n",
       nr,np,nz));
```

- An IC for eq. (8.1d), that is, eq. (8.2), is defined as the constant `T0`. The length of vector `u0` is declared with `rep` as `nr*nz = 6*11 = 66`, and this length informs the ODE integrator, `lsodes`, of the number of ODEs to be integrated.

```
#
# Initial condition
  u0=rep(0,nr*nz);T0=Ts;
  for(i in 1:nr){
  for(j in 1:nz){
    u0[(i-1)*nz+j]=T0;
  }
  }
  ncall=0;
```

The counter for the calls to `cryo_1` of Listing 8.1 is also initialized.

- The 66 ODEs are integrated by `lsodes`. Note the use of the IC vector `u0` to start the integration, the vector of output values of t, `tout`, and the ODE routine `cryo_1`. `y,times,func` are reserved names. `parms` for passing parameters to the ODE routine `cryo_1` is unused.

```
#
# ODE integration
  out=lsodes(y=u0,times=tout,func=cryo_1,parms=NULL);
  nrow(out)
  ncol(out)
```

- The number of calls to `cryo_1` is displayed at the end of the solution to give an indication of the effort to compute the numerical solution.

```
#
# Calls to ODE routine
  cat(sprintf("\n\n   ncall = %5d\n\n",ncall));
```

- Six 2D arrays are declared for the numerical solution at $r = 0, 1, \ldots, 5$.

```
#
# Plot z profiles
  T_zplot1=matrix(0,nrow=nz,ncol=nout);
  T_zplot2=matrix(0,nrow=nz,ncol=nout);
  T_zplot3=matrix(0,nrow=nz,ncol=nout);
```

```
T_zplot4=matrix(0,nrow=nz,ncol=nout);
T_zplot5=matrix(0,nrow=nz,ncol=nout);
T_zplot6=matrix(0,nrow=nz,ncol=nout);
```

These arrays have the numerical solution $T(r, z, t)$ as a function of z, t (with dimensions `nz,nout`).

- The numerical solution in `out` (from `lsodes`) is placed in the six arrays with two `for`'s that step through t and z.

```
for(it in 1:nout){
  for(j in 1:nz){
    T_zplot1[j,it]=out[it,      j+1];
    T_zplot2[j,it]=out[it,   nz+j+1];
    T_zplot3[j,it]=out[it,2*nz+j+1];
    T_zplot4[j,it]=out[it,3*nz+j+1];
    T_zplot5[j,it]=out[it,4*nz+j+1];
    T_zplot6[j,it]=out[it,5*nz+j+1];
  }
```

Note the offset of 1, for example, `j+1`, because the first position in the second dimension of `out` has the values of t.

- $T(r = 0, z = z_p, t) = T_p$ is set (with `j=np`) because this dependent variable is not computed with an ODE in `cryo_1` but is set by eq. (8.1e) (in general, the R ODE integrators do not return dependent variables that are not computed by the integration of an ODE).

```
    T_zplot1[np,it]=Tp;
    T_zplot1[1,it] =Ts;
    T_zplot2[1,it] =Ts;
    T_zplot3[1,it] =Ts;
    T_zplot4[1,it] =Ts;
    T_zplot5[1,it] =Ts;
    T_zplot6[1,it] =Ts;
}
```

Similarly, $T(r, z = 0, t) = T_s$ is set because the solution at $z = 0$ is not computed by the integration of ODEs (at $r = 0, 1, \ldots, 5$), but rather is set according to BC (8.3e). The final `}` concludes the `for` in t with index `it`. All of the `66` dependent variables are now in arrays `T_zplot1` to `T_zplot6` and can therefore be plotted.

- The plotting is done in two ways. For the first, the scaling of the vertical axis (for $T(r,z,t), r = 0, 1, \ldots, 5, t = 0, 30, \ldots, 120$) is performed automatically by `matplot`.

```
#
# Automatic vertical scaling for each plot
  par(mfrow=c(3,2));
  matplot(x=z,y=T_zplot1,type="l",xlab="z",
          ylab="T(r=0,z,t)",xlim=c(0,z[nz]),lty=1,
          main="T(r=0,z,t),t=0,30,...,120",lwd=2);
  matplot(x=z,y=T_zplot2,type="l",xlab="z",
          ylab="T(r=1,z,t)",xlim=c(0,z[nz]),lty=1,
          main="T(r=1,z,t),t=0,30,...,120",lwd=2);
  matplot(x=z,y=T_zplot3,type="l",xlab="z",
          ylab="T(r=2,z,t)",xlim=c(0,z[nz]),lty=1,
          main="T(r=2,z,t),t=0,30,...,120",lwd=2);
  matplot(x=z,y=T_zplot4,type="l",xlab="z",
          ylab="T(r=3,z,t)",xlim=c(0,z[nz]),lty=1,
          main="T(r=3,z,t),t=0,30,...,120",lwd=2);
  matplot(x=z,y=T_zplot5,type="l",xlab="z",
          ylab="T(r=4,z,t)",xlim=c(0,z[nz]),lty=1,
          main="T(r=4,z,t),t=0,30,...,120",lwd=2);
  matplot(x=z,y=T_zplot6,type="l",xlab="z",
          ylab="T(r=5,z,t)",xlim=c(0,z[nz]),lty=1,
          main="T(r=5,z,t),t=0,30,...,120",lwd=2);
```

A composite of six plots, that is, a matrix of plots with `3` rows by `2` columns is specified with `par(mfrow=c(3,2))`. Note the use of the grid in z, vector `z`, for the horizontal axis (designated as `x`). Also, the scaling of the horizontal axis of each plot is based on `z`, that is, `xlim=c(0,z[nz])`.

Each of the six 2D arrays with the solution plotted vertically as `y` has `nz` as a first (row) dimension which matches the dimension of `z`. This matching of the row dimensions for `x,y` is required by `matplot`. The 3×2 matrix of plots is in Fig. 8.2.

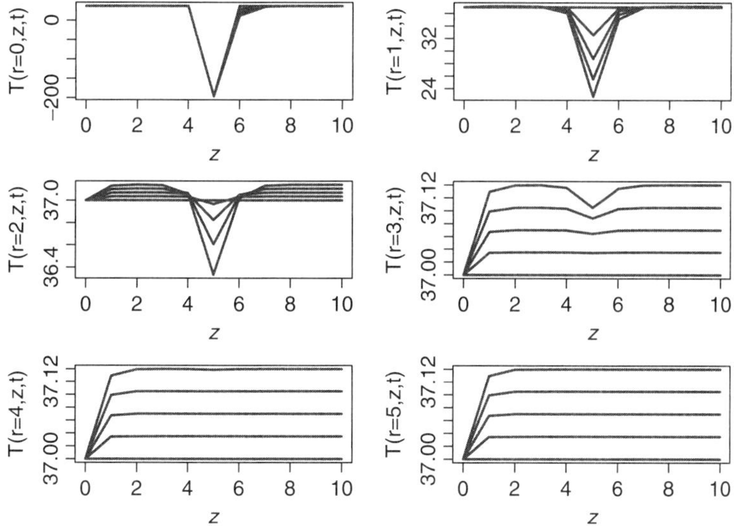

Figure 8.2 $T(r, z, t)$ versus z, $t = 0, 30, \ldots, 120$, $r = 0, 1, \ldots, 5$.

- While the automatic scaling of the vertical axis by `matplot` works as expected, it can give a misleading impression of the vertical position of the solution curves in the six plots. Thus, as a second way of plotting, the vertical scale is defined with `ylim=c(-200,40))` indicating the vertical scale for all six plots encompasses $-200 \leq T(r, z, t) \leq 40$. In this way, the six plots can be compared by inspection.

```
#
# Vertical scale set as -200 <= T <= 40
  par(mfrow=c(3,2));
  matplot(x=z,y=T_zplot1,type="l",xlab="z",
          ylab="T(r=0,z,t)",xlim=c(0,z[nz]),lty=1,
          main="T(r=0,z,t),t=0,30,...,120",lwd=2,
          ylim=c(-200,40));
  matplot(x=z,y=T_zplot2,type="l",xlab="z",
          ylab="T(r=1,z,t)",xlim=c(0,z[nz]),lty=1,
          main="T(r=1,z,t),t=0,30,...,120",lwd=2,
          ylim=c(-200,40));
  matplot(x=z,y=T_zplot3,type="l",xlab="z",
          ylab="T(r=2,z,t)",xlim=c(0,z[nz]),lty=1,
```

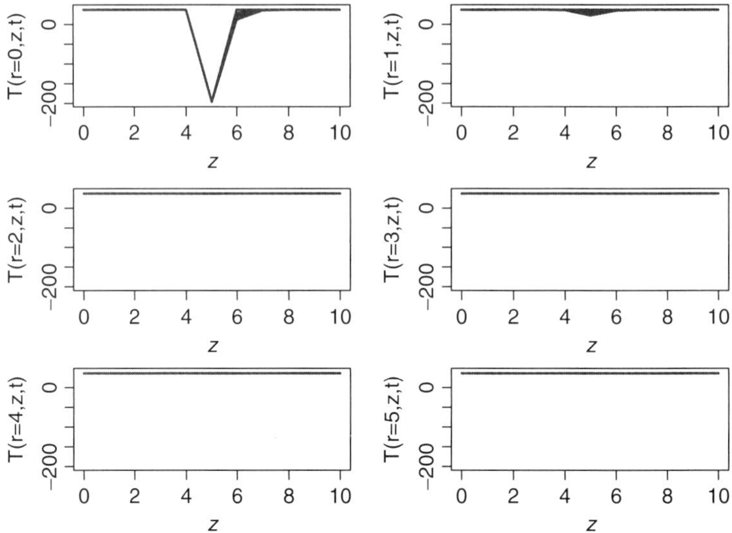

Figure 8.3 $T(r,z,t)$ versus $z, t = 0, 30, \ldots, 120, r = 0, 1, \ldots, 5$, $-200 \leq T(r,z,t) \leq 40$.

```
          main="T(r=2,z,t),t=0,30,...,120",lwd=2,
          ylim=c(-200,40));
matplot(x=z,y=T_zplot4,type="l",xlab="z",
          ylab="T(r=3,z,t)",xlim=c(0,z[nz]),lty=1,
          main="T(r=3,z,t),t=0,30,...,120",lwd=2,
          ylim=c(-200,40));
matplot(x=z,y=T_zplot5,type="l",xlab="z",
          ylab="T(r=4,z,t)",xlim=c(0,z[nz]),lty=1,
          main="T(r=4,z,t),t=0,30,...,120",lwd=2,
          ylim=c(-200,40));
matplot(x=z,y=T_zplot6,type="l",xlab="z",
          ylab="T(r=5,z,t)",xlim=c(0,z[nz]),lty=1,
          main="T(r=5,z,t),t=0,30,...,120",lwd=2,
          ylim=c(-200,40));
```

This completes the discussion of the main program in Listing 8.6. We next consider the output from the routines in Listings 8.1–8.6 (Figs. 8.2 and 8.3).

8.4 Numerical Output

The numerical output from Listing 8.6 is listed in Table 8.1.

TABLE 8.1 Numerical output from Listings 8.1–8.6.

```
nr =  6   np =  6   nz = 11

> nrow(out)
[1] 5
> ncol(out)
[1] 67

ncall =   103
```

We can note the following details about this output.

- The tip of the probe is at $r = 0$, $z_p = z_c/2$ (because `np` is at the midpoint value of `nz`).
- The solution array from `out` produced by `lsodes` has dimensions 5×67 corresponding to the five values $t = 0, 30, \ldots, 120$ and 66 ODEs with an additional 1 because `out` also includes t.
- The number of calls to `cryo_1` is quite modest.

The graphical output is in Figs. 8.2 and 8.3. We can note the following details about Fig 8.2.

- The solution $T(r, z, t)$ for eqs. (8.1)–(8.3) is displayed in 1D even though there are three independent variables.
- $T(r = 0, z, t)$ (top left figure for $r = 0$) indicates the probe tip temperature $T_p = -196$ at $z = z_p = 5$ cm. Elsewhere along the probe, the temperature is essentially $T(r = 0, z < z_p, t) = 37$. In other words, the cryogenic temperature is confined to a small region in the neighborhood of the probe tip as desired (to minimize the damage to normal or healthy tissue).
- In the $r = 0$ plot, there is a variation in temperature with t for $6 \le z \le 10$, whereas there is no corresponding variation in temperature for $0 \le z \le 4$. This lack of symmetry around $z = 5$ is due to the difference in BCs at $z = 0$ and $z = z_c$, that is,

BCs (8.3e,f). At $z = 0$ (BC 8.3e)), the temperature is maintained as $T_s = 37$ so that heat can flow into and heat the tissue near $z = z_p$ ($z < z_p = 5$). At $z = z_c = 10$, the no flux (no conduction) BC (8.3f) prevents any heat from flowing in (or out) so that the temperature near $z = z_p$ ($z > z_p = 5$) undergoes a cooling with increasing t. However, this latter effect is small and the temperature at $z = 6$ essentially remains at 37.

- The $r = 1$ plot also indicates the cooling by the probe tip (near $z = z_p = 5$). However, note the vertical scale which is approximately $23 \leq T \leq 37$ so the cooling is substantially less than that might be inferred (at $r = 1$). To emphasize this point, in Fig. 8.3, all of the vertical scales (of the six plots) are $-200 \leq T \leq 40$ to facilitate a visual comparison of the plots.
- The plots for $r = 2, 3, 4, 5$ indicate that the temperature remains close to 37 (again, note the vertical scales). In other words, the cooling is confined radially to less than 1 cm from the probe.
- The plots indicate that a steady state may not have been reached but using a t scale $0 \leq t \leq 240$ (4 min rather than 2) produces little change in the plots. Thus, it appears that the cooling does not spread in r and z with increasing t (mainly because of the temperature T_s at $z = 0$ and the metabolism Q_m in eq. (8.1d) that offsets the cooling).
- The plots have a rather kinky appearance because of the small number of points in r and z, 6 and 11, respectively, but increasing the number of points gives essentially the same semiquantitative results (limited spatial cooling) while smoothing the plots. Also, in this 2D problem, the number of ODEs increases rapidly with increasing numbers of grid points thereby requiring substantially more computation.

Fig. 8.3 with a common vertical scale $-200 \leq T \leq 40$ demonstrates that the cooling is confined to a small region or volume near the probe tip ($r = 0, z = z_p$) as desired.

This completes the discussion of the base case of eqs. (8.1)–(8.3). The model is based on the assumptions that can be investigated by experimenting with variations in the model as discussed next.

8.5 Variations in the Model

In the base case model, the probe is considered to be of a sufficiently small diameter that it is basically located at $r = 0$. The assumption could be investigated by placing the probe at $r > 0$, but the next grid point is at $r = 1$ with `nr=6` would describe a probe that is probably too large in diameter. Therefore, an increase in the number of radial grid points (a decrease in grid spacing in r) would be required to investigate the effect of probe diameter, or a nonuniform grid in r with points more closely spaced near $r = 0$ would be required. This extension of the model is not considered here but could be investigated by the reader.

Also, temperature variations along the exterior of the probe are not considered, that is, for $0 \leq z < z_p$. This effect could be investigated, for example, by setting the temperature along the probe to an assumed value in the same way that $T(r = 0, z = z_p, t)$ is specified in `cryo_1` (but $T_p = -196$ would not have to be used and a higher temperature would be more realistic). Again, the effect is not investigated here but could be accomplished with a straightforward modification of the $r = 0, 0 \leq z < z_p$ code in `cryo_1` of Listing 8.1. The result would be an indication of the tissue temperature distribution because of the increased cooling from the probe.

This discussion indicates one of the major advantages of the PDE model, that is, experimentation with the model by changing the parameters and equations is readily accomplished.

8.6 Summary

The model of eqs. (8.1)–(8.3) is intended as a presentation of several basic concepts.

- A PDE in 2D (two spatial variables and time).
- Variable coefficient ($1/r$).
- Nonlinear coefficients or functions ($C(T), k(T)$).
- Nonlinear nonhomogeneous source term ($Q_m(T)$).
- Dirichlet BCs ($z = 0$) and Neumann BCs ($r = 0, r = r_c, z = z_c$).
- Dependent variable explicitly defined at specific spatial points (rather than through the PDE), ($T(r = 0, z = z_c, t) = T_p$).
- MOL analysis based on library ODE integrators (`lsodes`) and explicit programming of finite difference approximations (in `cryo_1`).

The overall intention is to demonstrate the flexibility and generality of the numerical solution of PDE models, which is essentially unlimited in scope, and to suggest and illustrate concepts and procedures for PDE solution through a detailed example. The author welcomes enquiries and is pleased to suggest approaches to specific PDE applications and procedures.

References

[1] Deng, Z.-S., and J. Liu (2006), Numerical study of the effects of large blood vessels on three-dimensional tissue temperature profiles during cryosurgery, *Numerical Heat Transfer, Part A*, **49**, 47–67.

[2] Schiesser, W.E., and G.W. Griffiths (2009), *A Compendium of Partial Differential Equation Models*, Cambridge University Press, Cambridge, UK.

INDEX

Differential Equation Analysis in Biomedical Science and Engineering: Partial Differential Equation Applications with R, First Edition. William E. Schiesser.